W9-BWH-614

A Dictionary of Epidemiology

A DICTIONARY OF
EPIDEMIOLOGY

THIRD EDITION

Edited for the
International Epidemiological Association
by

John M. Last

Associate Editors

J. H. Abramson
Gary D. Friedman
Miquel Porta
Robert A. Spasoff
Michel Thuriaux

New York   Oxford   Toronto
OXFORD UNIVERSITY PRESS
1995

Oxford University Press

Oxford   New York
Athens   Auckland   Bangkok   Bombay
Calcutta   Cape Town   Dar es Salaam   Delhi
Florence   Hong Kong   Istanbul   Karachi
Kuala Lumpur   Madras   Madrid   Melbourne
Mexico City   Nairobi   Paris   Singapore
Taipei   Tokyo   Toronto

and associated companies in
Berlin   Ibadan

Published by Oxford University Press, Inc.,
200 Madison Avenue, New York, New York 10016

Oxford is a registered trademark of Oxford University Press

Library of Congress Cataloging-in-Publication Data
A dictionary of epidemiology / edited for the International
Epidemiological Association by John M. Last ; associate editors,
J. H. Abramson . . . [et al.].—3rd ed.
p.   cm. Includes bibliographical references.
ISBN 0-19-509667-3 (cloth).—ISBN 0-19-509668-1 (paper)
1. Epidemiology—Dictionaries.   I. Last, John M., 1926–
II. Abramson, J. H. (Joseph Herbert), 1924–   III. International
Epidemiological Association.
[DNLM: 1. Epidemiology—dictionaries.   WA 13 D553 1995]
RA651.D53   1995
614.4'03—dc20
DNLM/DLC
for Library of Congress   94-23361

2 4 6 8 9 7 5 3 1

Printed in the United States of America
on acid-free paper

Foreword

It is a great pleasure to introduce the third edition of the Dictionary of Epidemiology, sponsored by the International Epidemiological Association.

Epidemiological studies have been increasing worldwide for several decades; the rise of clinical epidemiology has made the field even wider. Basic scientists in pursuit of cause-effect relationships also are interested in the concepts and methods of epidemiology. Under these circumstances, definition of some terms needed to be modified or clarified, and the whole vocabulary of the relevant fields of biosciences has continued to expand.

John Last and his colleagues have reviewed all the terms in the dictionary, revising some of them appropriately; expanding some and dropping others; and adding many new terms from the relevant biomedical sciences. They deserve praise and admiration for the insight and devotion that they have brought to the task.

I hope not only epidemiologists and public health workers but also biologists and biomedical scientists in other fields will find it useful to keep this dictionary at hand and make the best use of it toward attaining our common goal of good-quality health for all.

Kunio Aoki, MD
President, International Epidemiological Association

Preface

This edition is a substantial revision. It contains almost 300 new entries and a similar number of revised definitions. In July 1993, I distributed about 200 candidate definitions to most of the editors listed in the second edition and to 75 other correspondents. In November 1993, I sent a revised list to 85 who had reacted to this material and to many former editors. In April 1994, I asked five of these, the Associate Editors of this edition, to review a further revision; while they were doing this, I added about 50 more items. Thus this edition is the combined work of a large team—though I accept all the blame for its defects. There is improved coverage of infectious disease epidemiology and control, health promotion, genetics, informatics, health economics, and biomedical ethics. It is difficult to decide where to set the boundaries around what we call "epidemiology." Admitting some terms at the interface between epidemiology and other disciplines is justified by the wide use of this dictionary outside the English-speaking nations: contributors who do not have English as their first language encouraged me to expand the horizons in this way. I deleted the "potted biographies" with mixed feelings; but the dates of many historically important and some contemporary epidemiologists survive in definitions associated with their names.

Ottawa   J. M. L.
September 1994

From the Preface to the Second Edition

This dictionary is intended for all who are interested in epidemiology, especially those who are beginning to study the subject, those whose first language is not English, and those from other fields who need to know the terms epidemiologists use.

Like all rapidly expanding sciences, epidemiology has been confounded by the proliferation of words and phrases to describe its concepts, principles, methods, and procedures. The creation of new terms and disagreement about the meaning of old ones can confuse beginners and established epidemiologists alike.

The dictionary is not an index of permitted and proscribed usage. I hope that it is authoritative without being authoritarian. Where synonyms exist, the definition appears under the most commonly used of these, but preference for one term over another is not necessarily implied. In a few instances, the use of a term is deprecated. Some terms that are properly described as slang or jargon have been included because they are widely used and their meaning is not always clear from the context. Murphy's description of jargon is worth recalling: "obscure and/or pretentious language, circumlocutions, invented meanings, and pomposity delighted in for its own sake."

All lay and technical vocabularies contain acronyms; epidemiology has its fair share. By convention, acronyms are spelt out the first time they appear in a text, and, if they are numerous, considerate editors sometimes supply a glossary, or at least list the acronyms along with the words for which they stand in an index. Although this dictionary is not the place for extensive mention of acronyms, a few appear here.

Eponyms, the attachment of personal or place names to concepts, diseases, methods, or specific studies, also occur often enough in published papers and books for us to recognize that beginners need some guidance to the meaning of those most widely used.

The compilers of dictionaries must exercise the greatest care in the choice of words and in their arrangement. Most entries in this dictionary have been repeatedly discussed with many contributors, and in nearly all instances the wording has been agreed upon by all; on the rare occasions when agreement eluded us, the final decision was mine alone. Therefore, I accept full responsibility for the deficiencies in the finished product.

J. M. L.

Acknowledgments

First I thank the International Epidemiological Association for entrusting to me the enjoyable task of compiling and revising this dictionary. I began preliminary work on this revision during a period as a scholar in residence at the Rockefeller Foundation Study and Conference Center, the Villa Serbelloni at Bellagio, Italy, in November–December 1992. (It was light relief from the main purpose of that scholarship, work on a book about ethical issues in epidemiology.) I thank the Rockefeller Foundation for this support. I thank the University of Ottawa and the Royal College of Physicians and Surgeons of Canada for mailing privileges and for the use of facsimile, word processing, and photocopying facilities.

The list of contributors is incomplete. When the second edition of the dictionary was published in 1988, I began to record the comments of colleagues. Some of these comments and the names of those who made them were lost when an annotated copy of the second edition disappeared from my office at the University of Ottawa. Other suggestions came from people at crowded seminars in Australia, Canada, New Zealand, and the United States. I thank these unnamed collaborators, as well as those on the accompanying list, on behalf of all who find this dictionary useful. I thank Jeffrey House of Oxford University Press for much encouragement, Stanley George for excellent manuscript editorial work, and Heidi Thaens for meticulous technical editing. Finally, I thank Wendy for help with proofreading and for sustaining me while I worked on this revision.

J. M. L.

Contributors

IBRAHIM ABDELNOUR
Damascus, Syria

JOE H. ABRAMSON
Jerusalem, Israel

ASRI ADISASMITA
Jakarta, Indonesia

KUNIO AOKI
Nagoya, Japan

JOHN C. BAILAR III
Montreal, Quebec, Canada

RENALDO N. BATTISTA
Montreal, Quebec, Canada

ROBERT BEAGLEHOLE
Auckland, New Zealand

NICHOLAS BIRKETT
Ottawa, Ontario, Canada

DANKMAR BÖHNING
Berlin, Germany

JEAN-FRANÇOIS BOIVIN
Montreal, Quebec, Canada

KNUT BORCH-JOHNSON
Copenhagen, Denmark

BEVERLEY CARLSON
New York, NY, USA

ROBERT M. CASTELLAN
Morgantown, WV, USA

WILLARD CATES, JR.
Atlanta, GA, USA

N. S. DEODHAR
Pune, India

THEODORE C. DOEGE
Chicago, IL, USA

DANIEL DORLING
Newcastle, England, UK

ROBERT M. DOUGLAS
Canberra, ACT, Australia

JOHN H. DUFFUS
Edinburgh, Scotland, UK

J. MARK ELWOOD
Dunedin, New Zealand

J. WALTER EWING
Barrie, Ontario, Canada

ALVAN R. FEINSTEIN
New Haven, CT, USA

CHARLES DU V. FLOREY
Dundee, Scotland, UK

EDUARDO L. FRANCO
Laval, Quebec, Canada

GARY D. FRIEDMAN
Oakland, CA, USA

JOHN W. FRANK
Toronto, Ontario, Canada

PHILIPPE GRANDJEAN
Odense, Denmark

CHARLES GUEST
Adelaide, SA, Australia

JEAN-PIERRE HABICHT
Ithaca, NY, USA

PHILIP F. HALL
Winnipeg, Manitoba, Canada

JØRGEN HILDEN
Copenhagen, Denmark

ALAN R. HINMAN
Atlanta, GA, USA

WALTER W. HOLLAND
London, England, UK

C. D'ARCY HOLMAN
Perth, WA, Australia

ERNEST B. HOOK
Berkeley, CA, USA

ANDREW HORNBLOW
Christchurch, New Zealand

PETER F. HOWARD
Brisbane, QLD, Australia

JAMES M. HUGHES
Atlanta, GA, USA

LESLIE M. IRWIG
Sydney, NSW, Australia

KONRAD JAMROZIK
Perth, WA, Australia

MILOS JENICEK
Montreal, Quebec, Canada

JUAN JUXING
Tangshan, China

CHARLES KERR
Sydney, NSW, Australia

JOCELYN KEITH
Wellington, New Zealand

MUSTAFA KHOGALI
Beirut, Lebanon

TORD KJELLSTRÖM
Geneva, Switzerland

THOMAS R. KNAPP
Rochester, NY, USA

KLAUS KRICKEBERG
Paris, France

HENK LAMBERTS
Amsterdam, Netherlands

JOSÉ M. LANDAVERDE
La Paz, Bolivia

JOHN M. LAST
Ottawa, Ontario, Canada

AHMED M. A. MANDIL
Alexandria, Egypt

JOHN MCCALLUM
Canberra, ACT, Australia

IAN W. MCDOWELL
Ottawa, Ontario, Canada

ANTHONY J. MCMICHAEL
London, England, UK

SALAH MOSTAFA
Cairo, Egypt

L. CAYOLLA DA MOTTA
Lisbon, Portugal

CARLES MUNTANER
Bethesda, MD, USA

ENRIQUE NÁHERA
Seville, Spain

RAMA C. NAIR
Ottawa, Ontario, Canada

KIUMARSS NASSERI
Los Angeles, CA, USA

JOHN S. NEUBERGER
Kansas City, KS, USA

NORMAN D. NOAH
London, England, UK

PATRICIA O'CAMPO
Baltimore, MD, USA

GRAEME OLIVER
Carlton, Victoria, Australia

JORN OLSEN
Aarhus, Denmark

CHARLOTTE PAUL
Dunedin, New Zealand

DIANA B. PETITTI
Pasadena, CA, USA

PETER O. D. PHAROAH
Liverpool, England, UK

MIQUEL PORTA
Barcelona, Spain

NURHAYATI PRIHARTONO
Jakarta, Indonesia

MATI RAHU
Tallinn, Estonia

José G. Rigau
San Juan, Puerto Rico

Aziza Salem
Cairo, Egypt

Clare Salmond
Wellington, New Zealand

George Salmond
Wellington, New Zealand

Rodolfo Saracci
Lyon, France

G. T. Satyavati
New Delhi, India

Andreu Segura
Barcelona, Spain

Thomas Shanks
San Diego, CA, USA

Peter Singer
Toronto, Ontario, Canada

Robert A. Spasoff
Ottawa, Ontario, Canada

Gregory J. Stoddard
Sandy, UT, USA

Larry Svenson
Edmonton, Alberta, Canada

Mervyn Susser
New York, NY, USA

Susan Tamblyn
Stratford, Ontario, Canada

José A. Tapia
Washington, DC, USA

Lukman Hakim Tarigan
Jakarta, Indonesia

Steven B. Teutsch
Atlanta, GA, USA

Steven Thacker
Atlanta, GA, USA

Michel Thuriaux
Geneva, Switzerland

Claes-Göran Westrin
Uppsala, Sweden

Kerr L. White
Charlottesville, VA, USA

Donald T. Wigle
Ottawa, Ontario, Canada

Russell Wilkins
Ottawa, Ontario, Canada

Hiroshi Yanagawa
Tochigi-Ken, Japan

Some Frequently Used Acronyms

ACE	American College of Epidemiology
ACHR	Advisory Committee on Health Research (WHO)
ADELF	Association des Épidémiologistes de Langue Française
AIDS	Acquired immunodeficiency syndrome
ANOVA	Analysis of variance
APHA	American Public Health Association
CDC	Centers for Disease Control and Prevention (of the United States Public Health Service)
CFR	Crude fertility rate, Case fatality rate
CIOMS	Council for International Organizations of the Medical Sciences
COPHC	Community-oriented primary health care
DALYs	Disability-adjusted life years
DFLE	Disability-free life expectancy
DSM-IV	*Diagnostic and Statistical Manual,* 4th ed. (of the American Psychiatric Association)
EC, EU	European Community, European Union
ELISA	Enzyme-linked immunosorbent assay
EIS	Epidemic Intelligence Service (US)
ENEE	European Network for Education in Epidemiology
EPA	Environmental Protection Agency (US)
EPI	Expanded Programme on Immunization (WHO/UNICEF)
EUPHA	European Public Health Association
GDP	Gross domestic product
GEENET	Global Environmental Epidemiology Network
GNP	Gross national product
GOBI/FFF	Growth monitoring, oral rehydration, breast feeding, immunization, family planning, food production, female education (WHO/UNICEF, World Bank)
GPA	Global Programme on AIDS (WHO)
HIV	Human immunodeficiency virus
IARC	International Agency for Research on Cancer

ICD-10	International Statistical Classification of Diseases and Related Health Problems, 10th Rev.
ICIDH	International Classification of Impairments, Disabilities and Handicaps
ICRC	International Commission of the Red Cross, Red Crescent
IEA	International Epidemiological Association
IGO	Intergovernmental organization (e.g., UN agencies)
IMR	Infant mortality rate
INSERM	Institut national de la santé et de la recherche médicale (France)
ISEE	International Society for Environmental Epidemiology
IUPAC	International Union of Pure and Applied Chemistry
KAP	Knowledge, attitudes, practice (of contraception)
MMR	Maternal mortality rate
MMWR	*Morbidity and Mortality Weekly Reports*
MRC	Medical Research Council (UK, Canada, other countries)
NCHS	National Center for Health Statistics (US)
NGO	Nongovernmental organization
NHANES	National Health and Nutrition Examination Survey (of NCHS)
NHMRC	National Health and Medical Research Council (Australia)
NIH	National Institutes of Health (US)
NIOSH	National Institute for Occupational Safety and Health (US)
ODA	Official development assistance
OECD	Organization for Economic Cooperation and Development
OPCS	Office of Population Censuses and Surveys (UK)
PAHO	Pan-American Health Organization
PATH	Programme for Appropriate Technology in Health
PHC	Primary Health Care
PMR	Perinatal mortality rate
PYLL	Potential years of life lost
QALE	Quality-adjusted life expectancy
QALYs	Quality-adjusted life years
RCT	Randomized controlled trial, Randomized clinical trial
REVES	Réseau espérances de vie en santé ([International] Network on health expectancy)
SEE	Sociedad Española de Epidemiología
SEER	Surveillance, epidemiology and end results (a program of the US National Cancer Institute)
SER	Society for Epidemiologic Research
UICC	Unione International Contre le Cancer (International Union for the Control of Cancer)
UN	United Nations

UNDP	United Nations Development Programme
UNEP	United Nations Environmental Programme
UNFPA	United Nations Fund for Population Activities
UNHCR	United Nations High Commission for Refugees
UNICEF	United Nations Children's Fund
USPHS	United States Public Health Service
WER	*Weekly Epidemiological Record* (published by WHO)
WHA	World Health Assembly
WHO	World Health Organization
YPLL	Years of potential life lost
ZPG	Zero population growth

A Dictionary of Epidemiology

A

ABORTION RATE The estimated annual number of abortions per 1000 women of reproductive age (usually defined as ages 15–44).

ABORTION RATIO The estimated number of abortions per 100 live births in a given year.

ABSCISSA The distance along the horizontal coordinate, or x axis, of a point P from the vertical or y axis of a graph. See also AXIS, GRAPH, ORDINATE.

ABSOLUTE POVERTY LEVEL Income level below which a minimum nutritionally adequate diet plus essential nonfood requirements is not affordable. (Source: UNICEF.)

ABSOLUTE RISK The observed or calculated probability of an event in a population under study, as contrasted with the relative risk. Sometimes this term is wrongly used as a synonym for ATTRIBUTABLE FRACTION, EXCESS RISK, or RISK DIFFERENCE.

ACCELERATED FAILURE-TIME MODEL A survival model in which exposure (or treatment) leads to alteration of the course of the disease. If the probability of being alive at time t is $S_0(t)$ under unexposed circumstances, then the probability for an exposed individual is

$$S(t) = S_0 (t/\gamma)$$

where γ is a measure of how much the course is altered. Thus if γ is 0.25, the course of the condition is four times as long as under conditions of nonexposure. Contrast PROPORTIONATE HAZARDS MODEL, in which the time pattern is fixed but the instantaneous mortality hazard is changed by exposure.

ACCEPTABLE RISK The risk that has minimal detrimental effects or for which the benefits outweigh the potential hazards. Epidemiologic study has provided data for calculation of risks associated with many medical procedures and also with occupational and environmental exposures; these data are used, for instance, in CLINICAL DECISION ANALYSIS.

ACCEPTANCE SAMPLING (Syn: stop-or-go sampling) Sampling method that requires division of the "universe" population into groups or batches as they pass a specified time point (e.g., age) followed by sampling of individuals within the sampled groups.

ACCIDENT An unanticipated event, commonly leading to injury, in traffic, the workplace, or a domestic or recreational setting. Epidemiologic studies have demonstrated that the risk of accidents is often predictable; they are therefore preventable.

ACCURACY The degree to which a measurement or an estimate based on measurements represents the true value of the attribute that is being measured. See also MEASUREMENT, TERMINOLOGY OF.

ACQUAINTANCE NETWORK Group of persons in contact or communication among whom transmission of an infectious agent and of knowledge, behavior, and values is possible and whose social interaction may have health implications. See also TRANSMISSION OF INFECTION.

ACQUIRED IMMUNODEFICIENCY SYNDROME (Syn: acquired immune deficiency syndrome) (AIDS) The late clinical stage of infection with HUMAN IMMUNODEFICIENCY VIRUS, recognized as a distinct syndrome in 1981. The surveillance definition[1] includes HIV-infected persons who have fewer than 200 CD4+ T-lymphocytes per μL, or a CD4+ T-lymphocyte percentage of total lymphocytes of less than 14%, accompanied by any of 26 clinical conditions (opportunistic infection, Kaposi's sarcoma, wasting syndrome, pulmonary tuberculosis, recurrent pneumonia, invasive cervical cancer, etc.).

The opportunistic or indicator diseases associated with AIDS include certain protozoal and helminth infections, notably *Pneumocystis carinii* pneumonia and toxoplasmosis; fungal infections, notably candidiasis of esophagus, trachea, bronchi, or lungs and cryptococcosis, especially affecting the central nervous system; bacterial infections, notably with certain mycobacteria including *Mycobacterium tuberculosis;* viral infections, notably cytomegalovirus and herpes simplex; and cancer, notably Kaposi's sarcoma, lymphoma limited to the brain, and invasive carcinoma of the cervix.

[1] 1993 revised classification system for HIV infection and expanded surveillance case definition for AIDS among adolescents and adults. *MMWR* 1992; 41:RR-17.

ACTIVE LIFE EXPECTANCY See DISABILITY-FREE LIFE EXPECTANCY.

ACTIVITIES OF DAILY LIVING (ADL) SCALE A scale devised by Katz and others[1] to score physical ability/disability; used to measure outcomes of interventions for various chronic disabling conditions such as arthritis. The scale is based on scores for responses to questions about mobility, self-care, grooming, etc. This was the first widely used scale of this type; others, mostly refinements or variations of the ADL scale, have since been developed.

[1] Katz S, Ford, AB, Moskowitz, RW, Jackson, BA, Jaffe, MW. Studies of illness in the aged: The index of ADL, a standardized measure of biological function. *JAMA* 1963; 185:914–919.

ACTUARIAL RATE See FORCE OF MORTALITY.

ACTUARIAL TABLE See LIFE TABLE.

ACUTE

1. Referring to a health effect, brief; sometimes loosely used to mean severe.
2. Referring to exposure, brief, intense, or short-term; sometimes specifically referring to brief exposure of high intensity. See also CHRONIC.

ADAPTATION A heritable component of the phenotype that confers an advantage in survival and reproductive success. The process by which organisms adapt to environmental conditions.

ADDITIVE MODEL A model in which the combined effect of several factors is the sum of the effects that would be produced by each of the factors in the absence of the others. For example, if factor X adds x% to risk in the absence of Y, and if factor Y adds y% to risk in the absence of X, an additive model states that the two factors together will add $(x+y)$% to risk. See also INTERACTION; LINEAR MODEL; MATHEMATICAL MODEL; MULTIPLICATIVE MODEL.

ADJUSTMENT A summarizing procedure for a statistical measure in which the effects of differences in composition of the populations being compared have been minimized by statistical methods. Examples are adjustment by regression analysis and by standardization. Adjustment often is performed on rates or relative risks, commonly because of differing age distributions in populations that are being compared. The mathematical procedure commonly used to adjust rates for age differences is direct or indirect standardization.

ADULT LITERACY RATE The percentage of persons age 15 and over who can read and write. (Source: UNICEF.)

ADVERSE REACTION An undesirable or unwanted consequence of a preventive, diagnostic, or therapeutic procedure. See also SIDE EFFECT.

AETIOLOGY, AETIOLOGIC See ETIOLOGY, ETIOLOGIC.

AGE The WHO recommends that age should be defined by completed units of time, counting the day of birth as zero.

AGE DEPENDENCY RATIO See DEPENDENCY RATIO.

AGENT (OF DISEASE) A factor, such as a microorganism, chemical substance, or form of radiation, whose presence, excessive presence, or (in deficiency diseases) relative absence is essential for the occurrence of a disease. A disease may have a single agent, a number of independent alternative agents (at least one of which must be present), or a complex of two or more factors whose combined presence is essential for the development of the disease. See also CAUSALITY; NECESSARY CAUSE.

AGE-PERIOD-COHORT ANALYSIS See COHORT ANALYSIS.

AGE-SEX PYRAMID See POPULATION PYRAMID.

AGE-SEX REGISTER List of all clients or patients of a medical practice or service, classified by age (birthdate) and sex; provides denominator for calculating age- and sex-specific rates.

AGE-SPECIFIC FERTILITY RATE The number of births occurring during a specified period to women of a specified age group, divided by the number of person-years lived during that period by women of that age group. When an age-specific fertility rate is calculated for a calendar year, the number of births to women of the specified age is usually divided by the midyear population of women of that age.

AGE-SPECIFIC RATE A rate for a specified age group. The numerator and denominator refer to the same age group.

Example:

$$\text{Age-specific death rate (age 25-34)} = \frac{\text{Number of deaths among residents age 25-34 in an area in a year}}{\text{Average (for midyear) population age 25-34 in the area in that year}} \times 100,000$$

The multiplier (usually 100,000 or 1,000,000) is chosen to produce a rate that can be expressed as a convenient number.

AGE STANDARDIZATION A procedure for adjusting rates, e.g., death rates, designed to minimize the effects of differences in age composition when comparing rates for different populations. See also ADJUSTMENT, STANDARDIZATION.

AGGREGATION BIAS (Syn: ecological bias) See ECOLOGICAL FALLACY.

AGING OF THE POPULATION A demographic term, meaning an increase over time in the proportion of older persons in the population. It does not necessarily imply an increase in life expectancy or that "people are living longer than they used to." In the past, the principal determinant of aging in the population has been a decline in the birth rate: when fewer children are born than in prior years, the result, in the absence of a rise in the death rate at higher ages, has been an increase in the proportion of older persons in the population. In developed societies, however, mortality change is becoming a factor: little further mortality reduction can occur in the first half of life, so reductions are beginning to occur in the third and fourth quarters of life, leading to a rise in the proportion of older persons from this cause.

AIDS-RELATED COMPLEX (ARC) Cluster of symptoms/signs occurring in some cases of HIV infection, including two or more of the following: Fever > 38°C, weight loss, persistent diarrhea, fatigue, lymphadenopathy, night sweats, anemia, leukopenia, thrombocytopenia, low CD4 T-cell count.

AIRBORNE INFECTION A mechanism of transmission of an infectious agent by particles, dust, or DROPLET NUCLEI suspended in the air. See also TRANSMISSION OF INFECTION.

ALGORITHM Any systematic process that consists of an ordered sequence of steps with each step depending on the outcome of the previous one. The term is commonly used to describe a structured process, for instance, relating to computer programming or to health planning. See also DECISION TREE.

ALGORITHM, CLINICAL (Syn: clinical protocol) An explicit description of steps to be taken in patient care in specified circumstances. This approach makes use of branching logic and of all pertinent data, both about the patient and from epidemiologic and other sources, to arrive at decisions that yield maximum benefit and minimum risk.

ALLELE Alternative forms of a gene, occupying the same locus on a chromosome.

ALMA-ATA DECLARATION See HEALTH FOR ALL, PRIMARY CARE.

ALPHA ERROR See ERROR, TYPE I.

ALPHA LEVEL See SIGNIFICANCE.

AMBIENT Surrounding; pertaining to the environment in which events are observed.

AMES TEST Bioassay for mutagenesis, using bacteria as target, to detect and screen for potentially carcinogenic compounds.

ANALYSIS OF VARIANCE (ANOVA) A statistical technique that isolates and assesses the contribution of categorical independent variables to variation in the mean of a continuous dependent variable. The observations are classified according to their categories for each of the independent variables, and the differences between the categories in their mean values on the dependent variable are estimated and tested for statistical significance.

ANALYTIC STUDY A study designed to examine associations, commonly putative or hypothesized causal relationships. An analytic study is usually concerned with identifying or measuring the effects of risk factors or is concerned with the health effects of specific exposure(s). Contrast DESCRIPTIVE STUDY, which does not test hypotheses. The common types of analytic study are CROSS-SECTIONAL, COHORT, and CASE CONTROL. In an analytic study, individuals in the study population may be classified according to absence or presence (or future development) of specific disease and according to "attributes" that may influence disease occurrence. Attributes may include age, race, sex, other disease(s), genetic, biochemical, and physiological characteristics, economic status, occupation, residence, and various aspects of the environment or personal behavior. See also RESEARCH DESIGN.

ANECDOTAL EVIDENCE Evidence derived from descriptions of cases or events rather than systematically collected data that can be submitted to statistical tests. Anecdotal evidence must be viewed with caution but sometimes is useful to generate hypotheses.

ANIMAL MODEL Study in a population of laboratory animals that uses conditions of animals analogous to conditions of humans to model processes comparable to those that occur in human populations. See also EXPERIMENTAL EPIDEMIOLOGY.

ANTAGONISM Opposite of SYNERGISM. The situation in which the combined effect of two or more factors is smaller than the solitary effect of any one of the factors. In BIOASSAY, the term may be used to refer to the situation when a specified response is produced by exposure to either of two factors but not by exposure to both together.

ANTHROPOMETRY The technique that deals with the measurement of the size, weight, and proportions of the human body.

ANTHROPOPHILIC (adj.) Pertaining to an insect's preference for feeding on humans even when nonhuman hosts are available.

ANTIBODY Protein molecule formed by exposure to a "foreign" or extraneous substance, e.g., invading microorganisms responsible for infection, or active immunization. May also be present as a result of passive transfer from mother to infant, via immune globulin, etc. Antibody has the capacity to bind specifically to the foreign substance (antigen) that elicited its production, thus supplying a mechanism for protection against infectious diseases. Antibody is epidemiologically important because its concentration (titer) can be measured in individuals, and, therefore, in populations. See also SEROEPIDEMIOLOGY.

ANTIGEN A substance (protein, polysaccharide, glycolipid, tissue transplant, etc.) that is capable of inducing specific immune response. Introduction of antigen may be by the invasion of infectious organisms, immunization, inhalation, ingestion, etc.

ANTIGENIC DRIFT The "evolutionary" changes that take place in the molecular structure of DNA/RNA in microorganisms during their passage from one host to another. It may be due to recombination, deletion or insertion of genes, to point mutations, or to several of these events. This process has been studied in common viruses, notably the influenza virus.[1] It leads to alteration (usually slow and progressive) in the antigenic composition, and thus in the immunologic responses of individuals and populations to exposure to the microorganisms concerned. See also ANTIGENIC SHIFT.

[1] Palese P, Young JF. Variation of influenza A, B, and C viruses. *Science* 1982; 215:1468–1473.

ANTIGENIC SHIFT Mutation, i.e., a sudden change in molecular structure of DNA/RNA in microorganisms, especially viruses, that produces new strains of the microorganism. Hosts previously exposed to other strains have little or no acquired immunity. Antigenic shift is believed to be the explanation for the occurrence of strains of the influenza A virus associated with large-scale epidemic and pandemic spread. Antigenic shift is responsible for the susceptibility of host populations to a new strain of influenza virus. See also ANTIGENIC DRIFT.

ANTIGENICITY (Syn: immunogenicity) The ability of agent(s) to produce a systemic or a local immunologic reaction in the host.

APACHE Acronym for Acute Physiology and Chronic Health Evaluation, a scoring system used to predict the outcome of critical illness or injury. This system and its variations (APACHE II, etc.) assign scores for state of consciousness, eye movements, reflexes, and physiologic data such as blood pressure.

APGAR SCORE A composite index used to evaluate neonatal status by assigning numerical scores (0–2) to heart rate, respiration, muscle tone, skin color, and response to stimulation. Developed by Virginia Apgar (1909–1974) a US pediatrician/anesthetist. Low scores are associated with a poor prognosis.

ARBOVIRUS A group of taxonomically diverse animal viruses that are unified by an epidemiologic concept, i.e., transmission between vertebrate host organisms by bloodfeeding (hematophagous) arthropod vectors such as mosquitoes, ticks, sand flies, and midges. The term is a contraction of *arthropod-borne virus*.

The interaction of arbovirus, vertebrate host(s), and arthropod vector gives this class of infections several unique epidemiologic features. See VECTOR-BORNE INFECTION for definition of terms used to describe these features.

AREA SAMPLING A method of sampling that can be used when the numbers in the population are unknown. The total area to be sampled is divided into subareas, e.g., by means of a grid that produces squares on a map; these subareas are then numbered and sampled, using a table of random numbers. Depending upon circumstances, the population in the sampled areas may first be enumerated, then a second stage of sampling may be conducted.

ARITHMETIC MEAN The sum of all the values in a set of measurements, divided by the number of values in the set.

ARTIFICIAL INTELLIGENCE A branch of computer science in which attempts are made to duplicate human intellectual functions. One application is in diagnosis, in which computer programs are based upon epidemiologic analyses of data in hospital charts or other clinical records.

ASCERTAINMENT The process of determining what is happening in a population or study group, e.g., family and household composition, occurrence of cases of specific diseases; the latter is also known as case finding.

ASCERTAINMENT BIAS Systematic failure to represent equally all classes of cases or persons supposed to be represented in a sample. This bias may arise because of the nature of the sources from which persons come, e.g., a specialized clinic; from a diagnostic process influenced by culture, custom, or idiosyncracy; or, for example, in genetic studies, from the statistical chance of selecting from large or small families.

ASSAY The quantitative or qualitative evaluation of a hazardous substance; the results of such an evaluation.

ASSOCIATION (Syn: correlation, [statistical] dependence, relationship) Statistical dependence between two or more events, characteristics, or other variables. An association is present if the probability of occurrence of an event or characteristic, or the quantity of a variable, depends upon the occurrence of one or more other events, the presence of one or more other characteristics, or the quantity of one or more other variables. The association between two variables is described as positive when the occurrence of higher values of a variable is associated with the occurrence of higher values of another variable. In a negative association, the occurrence of higher values of one variable is associated with lower values of the other variable. An association may be fortuitous or may be produced by various other circumstances; the presence of an association does not necessarily imply a causal relationship. If the use of the term *association* is confined to situations in which the relationship between two variables is statistically significant, the terms *statistical association* and *statistically significant association* become tautological. However, ordinary usage is seldom so precise as this. The terms *association* and *relationship* are often used interchangeably.

Associations can be broadly grouped under two headings, symmetrical or noncausal (see below) and asymmetrical or causal.

ASSOCIATION, ASYMMETRICAL (Syn: asymmetrical relationship) The definitive conditions of asymmetrical associations are direction and time. Independent variable X must cause changes in dependent variable Y; the "causal" variable must precede its "effects." The likelihood of a true causal relationship is increased by presence of certain criteria, but the only absolutely essential criterion is that the cause must precede the effect. See HILL'S CRITERIA. See also CAUSALITY; EVANS'S POSTULATES; HENLE-KOCH POSTULATES.

ASSOCIATION, DIRECT Directly associated, i.e., not via a known third variable: $A \rightarrow B$. Refers only to causality.

ASSOCIATION, INDIRECT CAUSAL Two types are distinguished:

1. Association of a factor *C* with disease *A* only because both are related to a common underlying factor *B*.

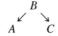

Alteration of factor *C* will not produce an alteration in the frequency to disease *A* unless an alteration in *C* affects *B*. It has been suggested that to avoid confusion with the alternative meaning of *indirect association,* this type should be called "secondary association."

2. Association of a factor *C* with disease *A* by means of an intermediate or intervening factor *B*.

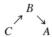

Alteration of factor *C* would produce an alteration in the frequency of disease *A*. To avoid confusion, this type should be called "indirect causal association."

ASSOCIATION, SPURIOUS A term, preferably avoided, used with different meanings by different authors. It may refer to artifactual, fortuitous, false secondary, or to all kinds of noncausal associations due to chance, bias, failure to control for extraneous variables, etc.

ASSOCIATION, SYMMETRICAL An association is noncausal if it is symmetrical, as in the statement $F = MA$ (force equals mass times acceleration). This is a noncausal, nondirectional expression of the mathematical relationship between the physical properties of force, mass, and velocity. If one side of the equation is changed, then the other must also change to maintain equilibrium.

Although epidemiologists are usually most interested in asymmetrical statements that have direction, the symmetrical equation can be useful. For instance, prevalence can be expressed in terms of incidence and duration in the simple equation, $P = I \times D$. If two of these three elements are known, the third can be derived. See also SYMMETRICAL RELATIONSHIP.

ASSORTATIVE MATING Selection of a mate with preference (or aversion) for a particular genotype, i.e., nonrandom mating.

ASYMMETRICAL ASSOCIATION See ASSOCIATION, ASYMMETRICAL.

ASYMPTOTIC Pertaining to a limiting value, for example, of a dependent variable, when the independent variable approaches zero or infinity. See LARGE SAMPLE METHOD.

ASYMPTOTIC CURVE A curve that approaches but never reaches zero or infinity, e.g., an exponential or reciprocal exponential curve.

ASYMPTOTIC METHOD See LARGE SAMPLE METHOD.

ATTACK RATE The cumulative incidence of infection in a group observed over a period during an epidemic. This "rate" can be determined empirically by identifying clinical cases and/or by means of seroepidemiology. Because its time dimension is uncertain or arbitrarily decided, it should probably not be described as a rate. See also INFECTION RATE, MASS ACTION PRINCIPLE, REED-FROST MODEL, SECONDARY ATTACK RATE.

ATTRIBUTABLE BENEFIT Antonym of ATTRIBUTABLE RISK; a term that can be used when exposure is beneficial rather than harmful.

ATTRIBUTABLE FRACTION (AF) (Syn: attributable proportion) A term sometimes used to refer to the attributable fraction in the population, and sometimes to the attributable fraction among the exposed. See also ATTRIBUTABLE FRACTION (EXPOSED); ATTRIBUTABLE FRACTION (POPULATION).

ATTRIBUTABLE FRACTION (EXPOSED) (Syn: attributable proportion [exposed], attributable risk, etiologic fraction [exposed]). With a given outcome, exposure factor and population, the attributable fraction among the exposed is the proportion by which the incidence rate of the outcome among those exposed would be reduced if the exposure were eliminated. It may be estimated by the formula

$$AF_e = \frac{I_e - I_u}{I_e}$$

where I_e is the incidence rate among the exposed, I_u is the incidence rate among the unexposed; or by the formula

$$AF_e = \frac{RR - 1}{RR}$$

where RR is the rate ratio, I_e/I_u. It is assumed that causes other than the one under investigation have had equal effects on the exposed and unexposed groups.

ATTRIBUTABLE FRACTION (POPULATION) (Syn: attributable proportion [population], etiologic fraction [population], attributable risk). With a given outcome, exposure factor, and population, the attributable fraction among the population is the proportion by which the incidence rate of the outcome in the entire population would be reduced if exposure were eliminated. It may be estimated by the formula

$$AF_p = \frac{I_p - I_u}{I_p}$$

where I_p is the incidence rate in the total population and I_u is the incidence rate among the unexposed; or by the formula

$$\frac{P_e(RR - 1)}{1 + P_e(RR - 1)}$$

where RR is the rate ratio, I_e/I_u. It is assumed that causes other than the one under investigation have had equal effects on the exposed and unexposed groups.

ATTRIBUTABLE NUMBER The number of new occurrences of a specific outcome attributable to an exposure; it may be estimated using the formula

$$AN = \frac{I_e - I_u}{N_e}$$

where I_e is the incidence rate among the exposed, I_u is the incidence rate among the unexposed, and N_e is the number of persons in the exposed population. It is assumed that causes other than the one under investigation have had equal effects on the exposed and unexposed groups.

ATTRIBUTABLE RISK The rate of a disease or other outcome in exposed individuals that can be attributed to the exposure. This measure is derived by subtracting the rate of the outcome (usually incidence or mortality) among the unexposed from the rate among the exposed individuals; it is assumed that causes other than the one under investigation have had equal effects on the exposed and unexposed groups. Unfortunately, this term has been used to denote a number of different concepts, including the attributable fraction in the population, the attributable fraction among the exposed, the population excess rate, and the rate difference. Therefore, it should be defined carefully by all who use it. See also ATTRIBUTABLE FRACTION (EXPOSED); ATTRIBUTABLE FRACTION (POPULATION); POPULATION ATTRIBUTABLE RISK; POPULATION EXCESS RATE; RATE DIFFERENCE.

ATTRIBUTABLE RISK (EXPOSED) This term has been used with different connotations to denote the attributable fraction among the exposed and the excess risk among the exposed. See also ATTRIBUTABLE FRACTION (EXPOSED); RATE DIFFERENCE.

ATTRIBUTABLE RISK (POPULATION) This term has been used with different connotations to denote the attributable fraction in the population and the population excess risk. See also ATTRIBUTABLE FRACTION (POPULATION); POPULATION EXCESS RATE.

ATTRIBUTABLE RISK PERCENT Attributable fraction expressed as a percentage rather than as a proportion.

ATTRIBUTABLE RISK PERCENT (EXPOSED) This is the attributable fraction among the exposed, expressed as a percentage. See also ATTRIBUTABLE FRACTION (EXPOSED).

ATTRIBUTABLE RISK PERCENT (POPULATION) This is the attributable fraction in the population, expressed as a percentage. See also ATTRIBUTABLE FRACTION (POPULATION).

ATTRIBUTE A qualitative characteristic of an individual or item.

AUDIT An examination or review that establishes the extent to which a condition, process, or performance conforms to predetermined standards or criteria. Assessment or review of any aspect of health care to determine its quality; audits may be carried out on the provision of care, compliance, community response, completeness of records, etc. See also HEALTH SERVICES RESEARCH.

AUSTRALIA ANTIGEN Hepatitis B surface antigen (HBsAg); so-called because it was first identified in an Australian aborigine. HBsAg is a BIOMARKER for the prevalence of infection with the virus of hepatitis B.

AUTONOMY, RESPECT FOR In ethics, the principle of respect for human dignity and the right of individuals to decide things for themselves. In epidemiologic practice and research, this principle is central to the concept of INFORMED CONSENT. It can conflict with the need to protect the population from identified risks, e.g., risks related to contagious disease, and with the need for access to personally identifiable health-related data and information. See also CONFIDENTIALITY, PRIVACY.

AUTOPSY DATA Data derived from autopsied deaths, e.g., for study of natural history of disease and trends in frequency of disease. Autopsies are done on nonrandomly selected persons in the population and findings should therefore be generalized only with great caution.

AVERAGE Distribution of aggregate inequalities in a series among all the members of the series, so as to equalize them. In science, loosely, the arithmetic mean. In everyday speech, ordinary, usual, or normal. In Anglo-Saxon, the word meant a day's work given to the feudal lord. Kendall and Buckland's *Dictionary of Statistical Terms* (4th ed, 1982) has this to say: "A familiar but elusive concept. Generally an 'average' value purports to represent or to summarize the relevant features of a set of values; and in this sense the term would include the median and the mode. In a more limited sense an 'average' compounds all the values of the set, e.g., in the case of the arithmetic or geometric means. In ordinary usage, 'the average' is often understood to refer to the arithmetic mean." See also MEASURE OF CENTRAL TENDENCY.

AVERAGE LIFE EXPECTANCY See EXPECTATION OF LIFE.

AXIS

1. One of the dimensions of a graph. A two-dimensional graph has two axes, the horizontal or x axis and the vertical or y axis. Mathematically, there may be more than two axes, and graphs are sometimes drawn with a third dimension; the eye cannot comprehend more than three dimensions.

2. In NOSOLOGY, an axis of classification is the conceptual framework, e.g., etiologic, topographic, psychologic, sociologic. The International Classification of Disease, for example, is multiaxial; the primary axis is topographic (i.e., body systems); secondary axes relate to etiology, manifestations of disease, detail of sites affected, severity, etc.

B

BACKGROUND LEVEL, RATE The concentration, often low, at which some substance, agent, or event is present or occurs at a particular time and place in the absence of a specific hazard or set of hazards under investigation. An example is the background level of naturally occurring forms of ionizing radiation to which we are all exposed.

BAR DIAGRAM A graphic technique for presenting DISCRETE DATA organized in such a way that each observation can fall into one and only one category of the variable. Frequencies are listed along one axis and categories of the variable along the other axis. The frequencies of each group of observations are represented by the lengths of the corresponding bars. See also HISTOGRAM.

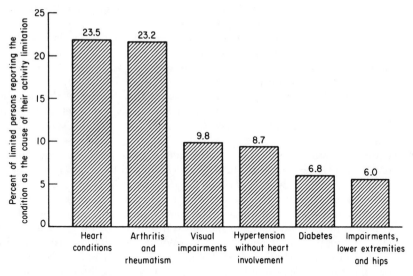

Bar chart, diagram. Activity limitation and self-reported conditions.
From Susser, Watson, Hopper, 1985.

BARRIER METHOD Contraceptive method that interposes a physical barrier between sperm and ovum.

BARYCENTRIC COORDINATES See PROFILE PLOT.

BASELINE DATA A set of data collected at the beginning of a study.

BASIC REPRODUCTIVE RATE (R_0) A measure of the number of infections produced, on average, by an infected individual in the early stages of an epidemic, when virtually all contacts are susceptible. (Some authors use the symbol Z_0 for basic reproductive rate.)

BAUD (rate) The unit of velocity of electronic transfer of data; 1 baud = 1 bit per second.

BAYES' THEOREM A theorem in probability theory named for Thomas Bayes (1702–1761), an English clergyman and mathematician; his *Essay Towards Solving a Problem in the Doctrine of Chances* (1763, published posthumously) contained this theorem. In epidemiology, it is used to obtain the probability of disease in a group of people with some characteristic on the basis of the overall rate of that disease (the prior probability of disease) and of the likelihoods of that characteristic in healthy and diseased individuals. The most familiar application is in CLINICAL DECISION ANALYSIS, where it is used for estimating the probability of a particular diagnosis given the appearance of some symptoms or test result. A simplified version of the theorem is

$$P(D|S) = \frac{P(S|D)P(D)}{P(S|D)P(D) + P(S|\overline{D})P(\overline{D})}$$

where D = disease, S = symptom, and $\overline{D}$ = no disease. The formula emphasizes what clinical intuition often overlooks, namely, that the probability of disease given this symptom depends not only on how characteristic that symptom is of the disease but also on how frequent the disease is among the population being served.

The theorem can also be used for estimating exposure-specific rates from case control studies if there is added information about the overall rate of disease in that population.

Some of the terms in the theorem are named. The probability of disease given the symptom is the *posterior probability*. It is an estimate of the probability of disease posterior to knowing whether or not the symptom was present. The overall probability of disease among the population or our guess of the probability of disease before knowing of the presence or absence of the symptom is the PRIOR PROBABILITY. The theorem is sometimes presented in terms of the odds of disease before knowing the symptom (*prior odds)* and after knowing the symptom (POSTERIOR ODDS).

BEHAVIORAL EPIDEMIC An epidemic attributable to the power of suggestion or to culturally determined behavioral patterns (as opposed to invading microorganisms or physical agents). Examples include the dancing manias of the Middle Ages, episodes of mass fainting or convulsions ("hysterical epidemics"), crowd panic, or waves of fashion or enthusiasm. The communicable nature of the behavior is dependent not only on person-to-person transmission of the behavioral pattern but also on group reinforcement (as with smoking, alcohol, or drug use). Behavioral epidemics may be difficult to differentiate from, or may complicate, outbreaks of organic disease, for example, due to contamination of the environment by a toxic substance.

BEHAVIORAL RISK FACTOR A characteristic or behavior that is associated with increased probability of a specified outcome; the term does not imply a causal relationship.

BENCHMARK A slang or jargon term, usually meaning a measurement taken at the outset of a series of measurements of the same variable, sometimes meaning the best or most desirable value of the variable. Because of uncertainty about meaning, the use of this term is not recommended.

BENEFIT Advantage or improvement resulting from an intervention.

BENEFIT-COST RATIO The ratio of net present value of measurable benefits to costs. Calculation of a benefit-cost ratio is used to determine the economic feasibility or success of a program.

BERNOULLI DISTRIBUTION The probability distribution associated with two mutually exclusive and exhaustive outcomes, e.g., death or survival; a Bernoulli variable is one that has only two possible values, e.g., death or survival. See also BINOMIAL DISTRIBUTION.

BERKSON'S BIAS A form of selection bias that leads hospital cases and controls in a case control study to be systematically different from one another.[1] This occurs when the combination of exposure and disease under study increases the risk of admission to hospital, leading to a systematically higher exposure rate among the hospital cases than the hospital controls; this, in turn, systematically distorts the odds ratio.

[1] Berkson J. Limitations of the application of fourfold table analysis to hospital data. *Biometrics Bull* 1946; 2:47–53.

BERTILLON CLASSIFICATION Jacques Bertillon (1851–1922) developed the first numerically based NOSOLOGY in which disease entities were arranged in chapters.[1] This was descended from a nosology proposed in 1853 by Marc d'Espigne and William Farr; Bertillon's classification was adopted at the International Statistical Institute (conference) in Chicago in 1893 and was the progenitor of the INTERNATIONAL CLASSIFICATION OF DISEASE (ICD).

[1] History and development of the ICD. ICD-10, Vol. 2, Geneva, Switzerland: WHO, 1993.

BETA ERROR See ERROR, TYPE II.

BIAS Deviation of results or inferences from the truth, or processes leading to such deviation. Any trend in the collection, analysis, interpretation, publication, or review of data that can lead to conclusions that are systematically different from the truth. Among the ways in which deviation from the truth can occur, are the following:

1. Systematic (one-sided) variation of measurements from the true values (syn: systematic error).
2. Variation of statistical summary measures (means, rates, measures of association, etc.) from their true values as a result of systematic variation of measurements, other flaws in data collection, or flaws in study design or analysis.
3. Deviation of inferences from the truth as a result of flaws in study design, data collection, or the analysis or interpretation of results.
4. A tendency of procedures (in study design, data collection, analysis, interpretation, review, or publication) to yield results or conclusions that depart from the truth.
5. Prejudice leading to the conscious or unconscious selection of study procedures that depart from the truth in a particular direction or to one-sidedness in the interpretation of results.

The term *bias* does not necessarily carry an imputation of prejudice or other subjective factor, such as the experimenter's desire for a particular outcome. This differs from conventional usage, in which *bias* refers to a partisan point of view.

Many varieties of bias have been described.[1]

[1] Sackett DL. Bias in analytic research. *J Chronic Dis* 1979; 32:51–63.

BIAS, ASCERTAINMENT See ASCERTAINMENT BIAS.

BIAS IN ASSUMPTION (Syn: conceptual bias) Error arising from faulty logic or premises or mistaken beliefs on the part of the investigator. False conclusions about the explanation for associations between variables. Example: Having correctly deduced the mode of transmission of cholera, John Snow concluded that yellow fever was transmitted by similar means. In fact, the "miasma" theory would have been a better fit for the facts of yellow fever transmission.

BIAS IN AUTOPSY SERIES Systematic error resulting from the fact that autopsies represent a nonrandom sample of all deaths.

BIAS, BERKSON'S See BERKSON'S BIAS.

BIAS DUE TO CONFOUNDING See CONFOUNDING.

BIAS, DESIGN See DESIGN BIAS.

BIAS, DETECTION See DETECTION BIAS.

BIAS DUE TO DIGIT PREFERENCE See DIGIT PREFERENCE.

BIAS IN HANDLING OUTLIERS Error arising from a failure to discard an unusual value occurring in a small sample or due to exclusion of unusual values that should be included.

BIAS, INFORMATION (Syn: observational bias) See INFORMATION BIAS.

BIAS DUE TO INSTRUMENTAL ERROR Systematic error due to faulty calibration, inaccurate measuring instruments, contaminated reagents, incorrect dilution or mixing of reagents, etc.

BIAS OF INTERPRETATION Error arising from inference and speculation. Sources of the error include (1) failure of the investigator to consider every interpretation consistent with the facts and to assess the credentials of each and (2) mishandling of cases that constitute exceptions to some general conclusion.

BIAS, INTERVIEWER See INTERVIEWER BIAS.

BIAS, "LEAD-TIME" See LEAD-TIME BIAS. See also ZERO TIME SHIFT.

BIAS, LENGTH See LENGTH BIAS.

BIAS, MEASUREMENT See MEASUREMENT BIAS.

BIAS, OBSERVER See OBSERVER BIAS. See also OBSERVER VARIATION.

BIAS IN THE PRESENTATION OF DATA Error due to irregularities produced by DIGIT PREFERENCE, incomplete data, poor techniques of measurement, or technically poor laboratory standards.

BIAS IN PUBLICATION See PUBLICATION BIAS.

BIAS OF AN ESTIMATOR The difference between the expected value of an estimator of a parameter and the true value of this parameter. See also UNBIASED ESTIMATOR.

BIAS, RECALL See RECALL BIAS.

BIAS, REPORTING See REPORTING BIAS.

BIAS, RESPONSE See RESPONSE BIAS.

BIAS, SAMPLING See SAMPLING BIAS.

BIAS, SELECTION See SELECTION BIAS.

BIAS DUE TO WITHDRAWALS A difference between the true value and that actually observed in a study due to the characteristics of those subjects who choose to withdraw.

BIAS, WORKUP See WORKUP BIAS.

BILLS OF MORTALITY Weekly and annual abstracts of christenings and burials compiled from parish registers in England, especially London, that date from 1538. Beginning in 1629, the annual bills were published and included a tabulation of deaths from plague and other causes. These were the basis for the earliest English vital statistics, compiled, analyzed, and discussed by John Graunt (1620–1674) in *Natural and Political Observations . . . on the Bills of Mortality* (London, 1662).

BIMODAL DISTRIBUTION A distribution with two regions of high frequency separated by a region of low frequency of observations. A two-peak distribution.

BINARY VARIABLE A variable having only two possible values, e.g., on or off, 0 or 1. See also BIT.

BINOMIAL DISTRIBUTION A probability distribution associated with two mutually exclusive outcomes, e.g., presence or absence of a clinical or laboratory sign, death or survival. The probability distribution of the number of occurrences of a binary event in a sample of n independent observations. The binomial distribution is used to model CUMULATIVE INCIDENCE rates and PREVALENCE RATE. The BERNOULLI DISTRIBUTION is a special case of the binomial distribution with $n = 1$.

BIOACCUMULATION Progressive increase in the amount or concentration of a chemical in an organism or in an organ or tissue when the rate of uptake exceeds the rate of excretion or metabolism. (Adapted from IUPAC Glossary.)

BIOASSAY The quantitative evaluation of the potency of a substance by assessing its effects on tissues, cells, live experimental animals, or humans.

Bioassay may be a direct method of estimating relative potency: groups of subjects are assigned to each of two (or more) preparations; the dose that is just sufficient to produce a specified response is measured, and the estimate is the ratio of the mean doses for the two (or more) groups. In this method, the death of the subject may be used as the "response."

The indirect method (more commonly used) requires study of the relationship between the magnitude of a dose and the magnitude of a quantitative response produced by it.

"BIOLOGICAL AGE" An attribute of body tissue that is relevant in pathogenesis, e.g., "age" of breast tissue, which develops after puberty, in relation to breast cancer risk.[1]

[1] Pike MC, Krailo MD, Henderson BE, et al: 'Hormonal' risk factors, 'breast tissue age' and the age-incidence of breast cancer. *Nature,* 1983; 303:767–770

BIOLOGICAL PLAUSIBILITY The criterion that an observed, presumably or putatively causal ASSOCIATION fits previously existing biological or medical knowledge. This judgment should be used cautiously since it could impede development of new knowledge that does not fit existing ideas.

BIOLOGICAL TRANSMISSION See VECTOR-BORNE INFECTION.

BIOMAGNIFICATION Sequence of processes in an ecosystem by which higher concentrations are attained in organisms at higher levels in the food chain. (Adapted from IUPAC Glossary.)

BIOMARKER, BIOLOGICAL MARKER A cellular or molecular indicator of exposure, health effects, or susceptibility. Biomarkers can be used to measure internal dose, biologically effective dose, early biological response, altered structure or function, susceptibility. See also MOLECULAR EPIDEMIOLOGY.

BIOMETRY (Literally, measurement of life) The application of statistical methods to the study of numerical data based on observation of biological phenomena. The term was made popular by Karl Pearson (1857–1936), who founded the journal *Biometrika.* The British biologist Francis Galton (1822–1911) has been described as the founder of biometry, but others—e.g., Pierre-Charles-Alexandre Louis (1787–1872)—preceded him.

BIOSTATISTICS Application of STATISTICS to biological problems. The term is considered by many biomedical scientists to mean the application of statistics specifically to medical problems, but its real meaning is broader.

BIRTH CERTIFICATE Official, legal document recording details of a live birth, usually comprising name, date, place, identity of parents, and sometimes additional information such as birth weight. It provides the basis for vital statistics of birth and birthrates in a political or administrative jurisdiction and for the denominator for infant mortality and certain other vital rates.

BIRTH COHORT See COHORT.

BIRTH COHORT ANALYSIS See COHORT ANALYSIS.

BIRTH INTERVAL Interval between termination of one completed pregnancy and the termination of the next.

BIRTH ORDER The ordinal number of a given live birth in relation to all previous live births of the same woman. Thus, 4 is the birth order of the fourth live birth occurring to the same woman. This strict demographic definition may be loosened to include all births, i.e., stillbirths as well as live births. More loosely, the ranking of siblings according to age, starting with the eldest in a family.

BIRTHRATE A summary rate based on the number of live births in a population over a given period, usually one year.

$$\text{Birthrate} = \frac{\begin{array}{c}\text{Number of live births to residents}\\\text{in an area in a calendar year}\end{array}}{\begin{array}{c}\text{Average or midyear population}\\\text{in the area in that year}\end{array}} \times 1000$$

Demographers refer to this as the *crude birthrate.*

BIRTH WEIGHT Infant's weight recorded at the time of birth and, in some countries, entered on the birth certificate. Certain variants of birth weight are precisely defined. Low birth weight (LBW) is below 2500 g. Very low birth weight (VLBW) is below 1500 g. Ultralow birth weight (ULBW) is below 1000 g. Large for gestational age (LGA) is birth weight above the 90th percentile. Average weight for gestational age (AGA) (Syn: appropriate or adequate): birth weight between 10th and 90th percentiles. Small for gestational age (SGA) (Syn: small for dates): birth weight below 10th percentile.

BIT Acronym for binary digit; the signal in computing. See also BYTE.

"BLACK BOX" (Jargon) A method of reasoning or studying a problem in which the methods, procedures, etc., as such are not described, explained, or perhaps even understood. Nothing is stated or inferred about the method; discussion and conclusions relate solely to the empirical relationships observed. An alternative definition is: A method of formally relating an input, e.g., quantity of a drug absorbed over a period or a putative causal factor, to an output, e.g., the amount of the drug eliminated in a given period, or an observed effect, without making detailed assumptions about the mechanisms that have contributed to the transformation of input to output within the organism (the "black box").

BLIND(ED) STUDY (Syn: masked study) A study in which observer(s) and/or subjects are kept ignorant of the group to which the subjects are assigned, as in an experiment, or of the population from which the subjects come, as in a nonexperimental study. When both observer and subjects are kept ignorant, we refer to a double-blind study. If the statistical analysis is also done in ignorance of the group to which subjects belong, the study is sometimes described as triple-blind. The intent of keeping subjects and/or investigators blinded, i.e., unaware of knowledge that might introduce a bias, is to eliminate the effects of such biases. To avoid confusion about the meaning of the word *blind,* some authors prefer to describe such studies as "masked."

BLOCKED RANDOMIZATION See STRATIFIED RANDOMIZATION. The analogue in a randomized experiment of individual matching in an observational study.

BLOT, WESTERN, NORTHERN, SOUTHERN Varieties of tests using electrophoresis, nucleic acid base pairing, and/or protein antibody interaction to detect and identify DNA or RNA samples. The *Southern blot*, named for its discoverer, E. Southern, is used to identify a specific segment of DNA in a sample. Molecular biologists named variations of the test for the points of the compass. The *Northern blot* detects and identifies samples of RNA. The *Western blot* is widely used in a test for HIV infection.

BODY BURDEN Total amount of a substance present in the body.

BODY MASS INDEX (Syn: Quetelet's index) Anthropometric measure, defined as weight in kilograms divided by the square of height in meters. This measure, suggested by the Belgian scientist Lambert Adolphe Jacques Quetelet (1796–1857), correlates closely with body density and skinfold thickness; in this respect it is superior to the PONDERAL INDEX.

BONFERRONI CORRECTION See MULTIPLE COMPARISON TECHNIQUES.

BOOTSTRAP A technique for estimating the variance and the bias of an estimator by repeatedly drawing random samples with replacement from the observations at hand. One applies the estimator to each sample drawn, thus obtaining a set of estimates. The observed variance of this set is the bootstrap estimate of variance. The difference between the average of the set of estimates and the original estimate is the bootstrap estimate of bias.

BOX-AND-WHISKERS PLOT (Syn: box plot) A graphical method of presenting the distribution of a variable measured on a numerical scale. The box-and-whiskers plot, sometimes called a box plot, is a graphic presentation of the information about a set of values contained in a STEM-AND-LEAF DISPLAY. The midpoint of the distribution is represented by a horizontal line; the values above and below this line are divided

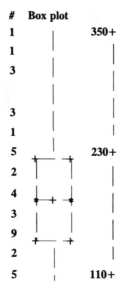

Box and whiskers plot. Four-week totals of reported cases of Meningococcal infections, United States, 1987–89. From Teutsch and Churchill, 1994.

into quartiles by horizontal lines (the "hinges" of the box) at the two quartiles nearer the midpoint; values beyond the hinges are represented by lines (the "whiskers") extending to the extreme value in each direction. Both the box-and-whiskers plot and the stem-and-leaf display were developed by the statistician John Tukey.[1]

[1] Tukey J. *Exploratory Data Analysis*. Reading, MA: Addison-Wesley, 1977.

BREAKPOINT In helminth epidemiology, the critical mean wormload in a community below which the helminth mating frequency is too low to maintain reproduction. A value exceeding the breakpoint of a wormload means that the wormload will increase until equilibrium is reached; a value less than or equal to the breakpoint means that the wormload will decrease progressively.

BYTE A group of adjacent bits, commonly 4, 6, or 8, operating as a unit for storage and manipulation of data in a computer. See also BIT.

C

CALIPER MATCHING see MATCHING.

CANADIAN MORTALITY DATABASE A large set of computer-stored death statistics; personal identifiers and causes of all deaths in Canada since 1950 have been computer-stored, and the death certificates have been preserved on microfiche. This data base and record linkage have been used in some important historical cohort studies. See also NATIONAL DEATH INDEX.

CANCER REGISTRY See REGISTER.

CAPTURE-RECAPTURE METHOD A method for estimating the prevalence of a condition in a population and the number of cases missed by various sources of ascertainment.[1,2] Data from several independent overlapping sample frames are compared to generate estimates of missing cases and the total number affected. The term originated in censuses of wild animals by capture-mark-release-recapture and was subsequently applied to human epidemiology. It is useful in studies of elusive populations, e.g., illicit drug users, street prostitutes. Compare SNOWBALL SAMPLING. A simple way to calculate an estimate of the total population at risk with two "captures" is to multiply the numbers and divide by the number caught in both captures. Prevalence rates are calculated in the same way.

[1] Wittes JT, Colton T, Sidel VW. Capture-recapture methods for assessing the completeness of ascertainment when using multiple information. *J Chronic Dis* 1974; 27:25–36.

[2] Laporte RE, Tull ES, McCarty D. Monitoring the incidence of myocardial infarctions; Applications of capture-mark-recapture technology. *Int J Epidemiol* 1992; 21:2:258–262.

CARCINOGEN An agent that can cause cancer. The International Agency for Research on Cancer (IARC) classifies carcinogens as follows:

1. *Sufficient evidence.* A positive causal relationship has been established between exposure and occurrence of cancer.
2. *Limited evidence.* A positive association has been observed between exposure to the agent, for which a causal interpretation is credible, but chance, bias, confounding cannot be ruled out.
3. *Inadequate evidence.* Available studies are of insufficient quality, consistency or statistical power to permit a conclusion regarding the presence or absence of a causal relationship.
4. *Evidence suggesting lack of carcinogenicity.* Several adequate studies covering the full range of doses to which humans are known to be exposed are mutually consistent in not showing a positive association between exposure to the agent and any studied cancer at any level of exposure.

Overall evaluation: Taking all the evidence into account, the agent is assigned to one of the following categories:

Group 1—The agent is carcinogenic to humans.

Group 2—At one extreme, the evidence for human carcinogenicity is almost sufficient (group 2A, probably carcinogenic); at the other, there are no human data but there is experimental evidence of carcinogenicity (group 2B, possibly carcinogenic).

Group 3—The agent is not classifiable as to its human carcinogenicity.

Group 4—The agent is probably not carcinogenic to humans.

CARCINOGENESIS The process by which cancer is produced. MOLECULAR EPIDEMIOLOGY can clarify aspects of this process. Several stages are recognized:

Initiation—The primary step of tumor induction; the irreversible transformation of a cell's growth-regulatory processes whereby the potential for unregulated growth is established, usually through genetic damage by a chemical or physical CARCINO-GEN.

Promotion—The second stage, in which a promoting agent induces an initiated cell to divide abnormally.

Progression—Transition of initiated promoted cells to a phase of unregulated growth and invasiveness, frequently with metastases and morphologic changes in the cancer cells.

CARRIER A person or animal that harbors a specific infectious agent in the absence of discernible clinical disease and serves as a potential source of infection. The carrier state may occur in an individual with an infection that is inapparent throughout its course (known as healthy or asymptomatic carrier) or during the incubation period, convalescence, and postconvalescence of an individual with a clinically recognizable disease (known as incubatory carrier or convalescent carrier). The carrier state may be of short or long duration (temporary or transient carrier or chronic carrier).[1]

[1] Adapted from Benenson AS, ed. *Control of Communicable Disease in Man,* 15th ed. Washington, DC: American Public Health Association, 1990.

CARRYING CAPACITY An estimate of the numbers of people that a nation, region, or the planet can sustain.

CASE In epidemiology, a person in the population or study group identified as having the particular disease, health disorder, or condition under investigation. A variety of criteria may be used to identify cases, e.g., individual physicians' diagnoses, registries and notifications, abstracts of clinical records, surveys of the general population, population screening, and reporting of defects such as in a dental record. The epidemiologic definition of a case is not necessarily the same as the ordinary clinical definition.

CASE, AUTOCHTHONOUS In infectious disease (malaria) epidemiology, a case of local origin. Literally, "native where it arises."

CASE-BASE STUDY A variation of the case control design in which the controls are drawn from the same STUDY BASE as the cases, regardless of their disease status.[1] Cases of the disease of interest are identified, and a sample of the entire base population (cases and noncases) forms the controls. This design allows estimation of the risk ratio because the exposure odds in the study base can be estimated.

[1] Kupper LL, McMichael AJ, Spirtas R. A hybrid epidemiologic study design useful in estimating relative risk. *J Am Stat Assoc* 1975; 70:524–528.

CASE-CASE STUDY A study in which cases with a specific characteristic such as a gene mutation are compared with other cases of the same condition without the characteristic, in order to identify etiologic factors specific to the subset of cases with this characteristic.[1]

[1] Taylor JA: Oncogenes and their application in epidemiologic studies. *Am J Epidemiol* 1989; 130:6–13

CASE-COHORT STUDY This analytic design compares the past histories of the cases of a condition of interest with the past histories of a sample of surviving noncases in the same cohort, matching the cases and noncases for duration of survival.[1] The case-cohort study design has the advantage of cost saving by using a sample of the original cohort. Contrast NESTED CASE CONTROL STUDY, in which cases and controls from the same cohort are not necessarily matched for duration of survival or follow-up.

[1] Wacholder S, Boivin JF. External comparisons with the case-cohort design. *Am J Epidemiol* 1987; 126:1198–1209.

CASE, COLLATERAL A case occurring in the immediate vicinity of a case that has been the subject of an epidemiologic investigation; a term used mainly in malaria control programs, equivalent to the term *contact* as used in infectious disease epidemiology.

CASE COMPARISON STUDY See CASE CONTROL STUDY.

CASE COMPEER STUDY See CASE CONTROL STUDY.

CASE CONTROL STUDY (Syn: case comparison study, case compeer study, case history study, case referent study, retrospective study) The observational epidemiologic study of persons with the disease (or other outcome variable) of interest and a suitable control (comparison, reference) group of persons without the disease. The relationship of an attribute to the disease is examined by comparing the diseased and nondiseased with regard to how frequently the attribute is present or, if quantitative, the levels of the attribute, in each of the groups. In short, the past history of exposure to a suspected RISK FACTOR is compared between "cases" and "controls," persons who resemble the cases in such respects as age and sex but do not have the disease or condition of interest.

Such a study can be called "retrospective" because it starts after the onset of disease and looks back to the postulated causal factors. Cases and controls in a case control study may be accumulated "prospectively"; that is, as each new case is diagnosed it is entered in the study. Nevertheless, such a study may still be called "retrospective" because it looks back from the outcome to its causes. The terms *cases* and *controls* are sometimes used to describe subjects in a RANDOMIZED CONTROLLED TRIAL, but the term *case control study* should not be used to describe such a study.

The terms *case control study* and *retrospective study* have been used most often to describe this method. Other terms also used are listed above. The concept of the case-control study is to be found in the works of P. C. A. Louis[1]; the first explicit description of the method is contained in a paper by William Augustus Guy, who reported his analysis of the relationship between prior occupational exposure and the occurrence of pulmonary consumption to the Statistical Society of London in 1843.[2] The evolution of the case control study thereafter has been described by Lilienfeld and Lilienfeld.[3] The first modern use of the method was a case control study of breast cancer reported by Lane-Claypon[4] in 1926; from that time onward, case control studies became increasingly popular and widely used. The design and analysis of case control studies have been much discussed.[5,6]

[1] Louis PCA. *Researches on Phthisis: Anatomical, Pathological and Therapeutical.* (Trans Wolshe WH). London: Sydenham Society, 1844.

[2] Guy WA. Contributions to a knowledge of the influence of employments on health. *J R Stat Soc* 1843; 6:197–211.

[3] Lilienfeld AM, Lilienfeld D. A century of case-control studies—Progress. *J Chronic Dis* 1979; 32:5–13.

[4] Lane-Claypon JE. A further report on cancer of the breast. *Rep Pub Hlth Med Subj* 32. London: HMSO, 1926.

[5] Breslow NE, Day NE. *Statistical Methods in Cancer Research: Vol 1. The Analysis of Case-Control Data.* Lyon: IARC, 1980.

[6] Wacholder S, McLaughlin JK, Silverman DT, Mandel JS: Selection of controls in case-control studies: I. Principles. *Am J Epidemiol* 1992; 135:1019–1028.

Wacholder S, Silverman DT, McLaughlin JK, Mandel JS. Selection of controls in case-control studies. II. Types of controls. *Am J Epidemiol* 1992; 135:1029–1041.

———: Selection of controls in case-control studies. III. Design options. *Am J Epidemiol* 1992; 135:1042–1050.

CASE-CROSSOVER DESIGN A variation of case control design that can be used when brief exposure causes a transient rise in the risk of a rare acute-onset disease.[1] Person-time incidence rates for persons in the group briefly exposed are compared with sample rates in the base population-time, e.g., to assess the effect of medication use on the short-term risk of myocardial infarction.

[1] Maclure M. The case-crossover design: A method for studying transient effects on the risk of acute events. *Am J Epidemiol* 1991; 133:144–153.

CASE FATALITY RATE The proportion of cases of a specified condition which are fatal within a specified time.

$$\text{Case fatality rate (usually expressed as a percentage)} = \frac{\text{Number of deaths from a disease (in a given period)}}{\text{Number of diagnosed cases of that disease (in the same period)}} \times 100$$

This definition can lead to paradox when more persons die of the disease than develop it during a given period. For instance, chemical poisoning that is slowly but inexorably fatal may cause many persons to develop the disease over a relatively short period of time, but the deaths may not occur until some years later and may be spread over a period of years during which there are no new cases. Thus, in calculating the case fatality rate, it is necessary to acknowledge that the time dimension varies: it may be brief, e.g., covering only the period of stay in a hospital; of finite duration, e.g., one year; or of longer duration still. The term *case fatality rate* is then better replaced by a term such as *survival rate* or by the use of a survivorship table. See also ATTACK RATE, SURVIVORSHIP STUDY.

CASE HISTORY STUDY

1. Synonym for CASE CONTROL STUDY.

2. In clinical medicine, a case report or a report on a series of cases.

CASE, IMPORTED In infectious disease (malaria) epidemiology, a case that has entered a region by land, sea, or air transport, in contrast to one acquired locally.

CASE, INDIGENOUS In infectious disease (malaria) epidemiology, a case in a person residing in the area.

CASE, INDUCED In malaria epidemiology, a case occurring in a person who has received a transfusion of blood containing malaria parasites; the term is generalizable to other conditions that can be transmitted in infected blood, e.g., HIV infection, hepatitis C.

CASE-MIX INDEX (CMI) A measure of the complexity of illness. Among hospital patients, it is based on the relative severity indexes assigned to a DIAGNOSIS-RELATED GROUP. A high CMI indicates a high proportion of complex cases and justifies higher rates of reimbursement in medical care insurance systems such as Medicare.

CASE REFERENT STUDY See CASE CONTROL STUDY.

CATASTROPHE THEORY A branch of mathematics dealing with large changes in the total system that may result from small changes in a critical variable in the system. An example is the sudden change in the physical state of water into steam or ice with rise or fall of temperature beyond a critical level. Certain epidemics, gene frequencies, and behavioral phenomena in populations may abide by the same mathematical rule. Herd immunity is an example. See also CHAOS THEORY.

CATCHMENT AREA Region from which the clients of a particular health facility are drawn. Such a region may be well or ill defined.

CAUSALITY The relating of causes to the effects they produce. Most of epidemiology concerns causality and several types of causes can be distinguished. It must be emphasized, however, that epidemiologic evidence by itself is insufficient to establish causality, although it can provide powerful circumstantial evidence.

A cause is termed "necessary" when it must always precede an effect. This effect need not be the sole result of the one cause. A cause is termed "sufficient" when it inevitably initiates or produces an effect. Any given cause may be necessary, sufficient, neither, or both. These possibilities are explained below.

Four conditions under which independent variable X may cause Y:

| | variable X may cause Y | |
	X is necessary	X is sufficient
1.	+	+
2.	+	−
3.	−	+
4.	−	−

1. X is necessary and sufficient to cause Y. Both X and Y are always present together, and nothing but X is needed to cause Y; $X{\to}Y$. For example, the measles virus is necessary to cause measles in an unimmunized individual or population.
2. X is necessary but not sufficient to cause Y. X must be present when Y is present, but Y is not always present when X is. Some additional factor(s) must also be present; X and $Z{\to}Y$. *Mycobacterium tuberculosis* is the necessary cause of tuberculosis but often is not a sufficient cause without poverty, poor nutrition, overcrowding, etc.
3. X is not necessary but is sufficient to cause Y. Y is present when X is, but X may or may not be present when Y is present, because Y has other causes and can occur without X. For example, an enlarged spleen can have many separate causes that are unconnected with each other; $X{\to}Y$; $Z{\to}Y$. Lung cancer can be caused by cigarette smoking, asbestos fibers, or radon gas.
4. X is neither necessary nor sufficient to cause Y. Again, X may or may not be present when Y is present. Under these conditions, however, if X is present with Y, some additional factor must also be present. Here X is a contributory cause of Y in some causal sequences; X and $Z{\to}Y$; W and $Z{\to}Y$. These relationships and the logic of causal inference are discussed in *Causal Inference*[1] and by Susser.[2] See also HILL'S CRITERIA.

[1] Rothman KJ, ed. *Causal Inference*. Chestnut Hill, MA: Epidemiology Resources, 1988.
[2] Susser MW. What is a cause and how do we know one? *Am J Epidemiol* 1991; 133:635–648.

CAUSATION OF DISEASE, FACTORS IN The following factors have been differentiated (but they are not mutually exclusive):

Predisposing factors are those that prepare, sensitize, condition, or otherwise create a situation such as a level of immunity or state of susceptibility so that the host tends to react in a specific fashion to a disease agent, personal interaction, environmental stimulus, or specific incentive. Examples include age, sex, marital status, family size, educational level, previous illness experience, presence of concurrent illness, dependency, working environment, and attitudes toward the use of health services. These factors may be "necessary" but are rarely "sufficient" to cause the phenomenon under study.

Enabling factors are those that facilitate the manifestation of disease, disability, ill-health, or the use of services or conversely those that facilitate recovery from illness, maintenance or enhancement of health status, or more appropriate use of health services. Examples include income, health insurance coverage, nutrition, climate, housing, personal support systems, and availability of medical care. These factors may be "necessary" but are rarely "sufficient" to cause the phenomenon under study.

Precipitating factors are those associated with the definitive onset of a disease, illness, accident, behavioral response, or course of action. Usually one factor is more important or more obviously recognizable than others if several are involved and one may often be regarded as "necessary." Examples include exposure to specific disease, amount or level of an infectious organism, drug, noxious agent, physical trauma, personal interaction, occupational stimulus, or new awareness or knowledge.

Reinforcing factors are those tending to perpetuate or aggravate the presence of a disease, disability, impairment, attitude, pattern of behavior, or course of action. They may tend to be repetitive, recurrent, or persistent and may or may not necessarily be the same or similar to those categorized as predisposing, enabling, or precipitating. Examples include repeated exposure to the same noxious stimulus (in the absence of an appropriate immune response) such as an infectious agent, work, household, or interpersonal environment, presence of financial incentive or disincentive, personal satisfaction or deprivation.

CAUSES OF DEATH See DEATH CERTIFICATE.

CAUSE-DELETED LIFE TABLE A life table constructed using death rates lowered by eliminating the risk of dying from a specified cause; its most common use is to calculate the gain in life expectancy that would result from the elimination of one cause.

CAUSE-SPECIFIC RATE A rate that specifies events, such as deaths, according to their cause.

CENSORING

1. Loss of subjects from a follow-up study; the occurrence of the event of interest among such subjects is uncertain after a specified time when it was known that the event of interest had *not* occurred; it is not known, however, if or when the event of interest occurred subsequently. Such subjects are described as *censored*. For example, in a follow-up study with myocardial infarction as the outcome of interest, a subject who has not had an infarct but is killed in a traffic crash in year 6 is described as censored as of year 6, since it cannot be known when, if ever, he might have had an infarct at a later year of follow-up. This is censoring by competing risk; other varieties include loss to follow-up and termination of the study. Examination of data for censoring requires the use of special analytic methods, such as life table analysis.

2. Observations with unknown values from one end of a frequency distribution, occurring beyond a measurement threshold. Left-censored data come from the left-hand or low end and right-censored data come from the right-hand or high end of the distribution.

CENSUS An enumeration of a population, originally intended for purposes of taxation and military service. Ancient civilizations such as the Romans conducted censuses;

Jesus of Nazareth was born in Bethlehem because Mary and Joseph had gone there to be counted in a Roman census. Census enumeration of a population usually records identities of all persons in every place of residence, with age, or birth date, sex, occupation, national origin, language, marital status, income, and relationship to head of household in addition to information on the dwelling place. Many other items of information may be included, e.g., educational level (or literacy), and health-related data such as permanent disability. A de facto census allocates persons according to their location at the time of enumeration. A de jure census assigns persons according to their usual place of residence at the time of enumeration.

CENSUS TRACT An area for which details of population structure are separately tabulated at a periodic census; normally it is the smallest unit of analysis of census tabulations. Census tracts are chosen because they have well-defined boundaries, sometimes the same as local political jurisdictions, sometimes defined by conspicuous geographical features such as main roads, rivers. In urban areas census tracts may be further subdivided, e.g., into city blocks, but published tables do not contain details to this level.

CENTILE See QUANTILES.

CESSATION EXPERIMENT Controlled study in which an attempt is made to evaluate the termination of an exposure to risk such as a living habit that is considered to be of etiologic importance.

CHAOS THEORY Branch of mathematics discovered by Edward Lorenz in 1963, dealing with events and processes that cannot be predicted by conventional mathematical theorems or laws because small, localized perturbations have widespread general consequences. Examples include long-range weather changes, turbulence in fast-flowing water. The unpredictable course of some epidemics and metastases in many kinds of cancer accord with chaos theory.

CHART The medical dossier of a patient. See also INFORMATION SYSTEM; MEDICAL RECORD.

CHECK DIGIT A single digit, derived from a multidigit number such as a case identification number, that is used as a screening test for transcription errors.

CHEMOPROPHYLAXIS The administration of a chemical, including antibiotics, to prevent the development of an infection or the progression of an infection to active manifest disease.

CHEMOTHERAPY The use of a chemical to treat a clinically recognizable disease or to limit its further progress.

CHILD DEATH RATE The number of deaths of children age 1–4 years in a given year per 1000 children in this age group. This is a useful measure of the burden of preventable communicable diseases in the child population.

CHILD MORTALITY RATE (Syn: Under-5 mortality rate) The United Nations Children's Fund (UNICEF) defines this as the annual number of deaths of children age under 5 years, expressed as a rate per thousand live births, averaged over the previous 5 years. This rate is preferable to the child death rate, which is more difficult to determine in communities where the age of young children may not be known precisely.

CHILD NUTRITION, MEASURES OF The United Nations Children's Fund (UNICEF) defines several aspects of infant and child nutrition:

Stunting A measure of protein-energy malnutrition, indicated by low height for age, failure to achieve expected stature.

Underweight A composite measure of protein-energy childhood malnutrition, indicated by low weight for age.

Wasting A measure of protein-energy malnutrition that occurs when a child's weight for height falls significantly below what is expected in the reference population; an indicator of current malnutrition.

CHI-SQUARE (χ^2) DISTRIBUTION A variable is said to have a chi-square distribution with K degrees of freedom if it is distributed like the sum of the squares of K independent random variables, each of which has a normal distribution with mean zero and variance one.

CHI-SQUARE (χ^2) TEST Any statistical test based on comparison of a test statistic to a chi-square distribution. The oldest and most common chi-square tests are for detecting whether two or more population distributions differ from one another; these tests usually involve counts of data, and may involve comparison of samples from the distributions under study, or the comparison of a sample to a theoretically expected distribution. The Pearson chi-square test is probably the best known; another is the MANTEL-HAENSZEL TEST. (Statisticians disagree about the terminal letter; most of those who contributed to the discussion of this entry prefer *chi-square* rather than *chi-squared*. Either usage is acceptable.)

CHOROPLETHIC MAP A method of mapping to display quantitative information, e.g., rates, in defined jurisdictions such as counties, states; an example is a color-coded atlas of cancer mortality.

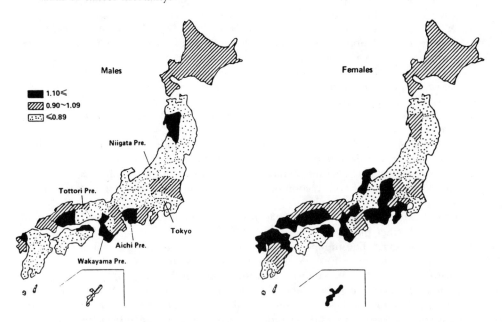

Choroplethic map. Regional differences of hip fracture incidence in Japan. From Hosoda et al., *Japanese Journal of Epidemiology*, 1992, 2:*Suppl* 2: S205–S213, with permission.

CHRISOMS This word, which appears in BILLS OF MORTALITY, means infants who die before formal baptism; therefore, the number recorded in Bills of Mortality can be used to estimate (albeit inaccurately) neonatal death rates in studies of historical demography and epidemiology.

CHRONIC 1. Referring to a health-related state, lasting a long time. 2. Referring to exposure, prolonged or long-term, often with specific reference to low intensity. 3. The US National Center for Health Statistics defines a "chronic" condition as one of 3 months' duration or longer.

CHRONOBIOLOGY The study of biological processes that possess periodicity, e.g., circadian rhythms, the menstrual cycle.

CLASS A term used in the theory of frequency distributions. The total number of observations made upon a particular variate may be grouped into classes according to convenient divisions of the variate range in order to make subsequent analyses less laborious or for other reasons. A group so determined is called a *class.* The variate values that determine the upper and lower limits of a class are called *class boundaries,* the interval between them is the *class interval,* and the frequency falling into the class is the *class frequency.* See also SET.

CLASS INTERVAL The difference between the lower and upper limits of a class.

CLASSIFICATION (Syn: categorization) Assignment to predesignated classes on the basis of perceived common characteristics. A means of giving order to a group of disconnected facts. Ideally, a classification should be characterized by (1) naturalness—the classes correspond to the nature of the thing being classified, (2) exhaustiveness— every member of the group will fit into one (and only one) class in the system, (3) usefulness—the classification is practical, (4) simplicity—the subclasses are not excessive, and (5) constructability—the set of classes can be constructed by a demonstrably systematic procedure.

CLASSIFICATION OF DISEASES Arrangement of diseases into groups having common characteristics. Useful in efforts to achieve standardization, and therefore comparability, in the methods of presentation of mortality and morbidity data from different sources. May include a systematic numerical notation for each disease entry.

Examples include the INTERNATIONAL CLASSIFICATION OF DISEASES (ICD) and the INTERNATIONAL CLASSIFICATION OF HEALTH PROBLEMS IN PRIMARY CARE (ICHPPC).

CLASS, SOCIAL A method of socially stratifying populations, e.g., according to education, income, or occupation. See also SOCIOECONOMIC CLASSIFICATION.

CLINICAL DECISION ANALYSIS Application of DECISION ANALYSIS in a clinical setting with the aim of applying epidemiologic and other data on probability of outcomes when alternative decisions can be made, e.g., surgical intervention or drug treatment for myocardial ischemia. Clinical decision analysis considers three aspects of the decision: choices (options available to the patient), chances (probabilities of outcome for each choice), and values (quantitative expression of the desirability of different outcomes).[1]

[1] Plume SK. Choices, chances, values. *Ann Thorac Surg* 1992; 53:373.

CLINICAL ECOLOGY The study of ENVIRONMENTAL HYPERSENSITIVITY.

CLINICAL EPIDEMIOLOGIST A practitioner of clinical epidemiology.

CLINICAL EPIDEMIOLOGY Epidemiologic study conducted in a clinical setting, usually by clinicians, with patients as the subjects of study. Paul[1] defined the term as "A marriage between quantitative concepts used by epidemiologists to study disease in populations and decision-making in the individual case which is the daily fare of clinical medicine." The most succinct modern definition may be "the application of epidemiologic principles and methods to problems encountered in clinical medicine."[2] Jenicek[3] suggests that the essential feature of clinical epidemiology is the direction of inference: classic epidemiology seeks to identify causes and measure risks of disease. Clinical epidemiology uses the information from classic epidemiology to aid decision making about identified cases of disease. The distinction between clinical epidemiology and CLINICAL DECISION ANALYSIS may be that the epidemiologist works with a defined population; clinical decision analysis can be applied to small numbers such as a clinical series of cases, even to a single patient (see N-OF-ONE STUDY). In some academic centers the adjective *clinical* can describe other disciplines. Thus *clinical economics* is the application of cost-benefit and cost-effectiveness analytic techniques in a clinical setting.

[1] Paul JR: Clinical epidemiology *J Clin Invest* 1938; 17:539–541.

[2] Fletcher RH, Fletcher SW, Wagner EH. *Clinical Epidemiology—the Essentials*. Baltimore: Williams & Wilkins, 1982.

[3] Jenicek M, Cléroux R. *Épidémiologie clinique (Clinométrie)*. Ste-Hyacinthe, Que: Edisem, 1985.

CLINICAL TRIAL (Syn: therapeutic trial) A research activity that involves the administration of a test regimen to humans to evaluate its efficacy and safety. The term is subject to wide variation in usage, from the first use in humans without any control treatment to a rigorously designed and executed experiment involving test and control treatments and randomization. Several phases of clinical trials are distinguished:

Phase I trial Safety and pharmacologic profiles. The first introduction of a candidate vaccine or a drug into a human population to determine its safety and mode of action. In drug trials, this phase may include studies of dose and route of administration. Phase I trials usually involve fewer than 100 healthy volunteers.

Phase II trial Pilot efficacy studies. Initial trial to examine efficacy usually in 200 to 500 volunteers; with vaccines, the focus is on immunogenicity, and with drugs, on demonstration of safety and efficacy in comparison to other existing regimens. Usually but not always, subjects are randomly allocated to study and control groups.

Phase III trial Extensive clinical trial. This phase is intended for complete assessment of safety and efficacy. It involves larger numbers, perhaps thousands, of volunteers, usually with random allocation to study and control groups, and may be a multicenter trial.

Phase IV trial With drugs, this phase is conducted after the national drug registration authority (e.g., the Food and Drug Administration in the United States) has approved the drug for distribution or marketing. Phase IV trials may include research designed to explore a specific pharmacologic effect, to establish the incidence of adverse reactions, or to determine the effects of long-term use. Ethical review is required for phase IV clinical trials, but not for routine POSTMARKETING SURVEILLANCE.

See also COMMUNITY TRIAL.

CLINIMETRICS Feinstein,[1] who coined this term, defines it as the domain concerned with indexes, rating scales, and other expressions that are used to describe or measure symptoms, physical signs, and other distinctly clinical phenomena in clinical medicine. Such measurements, of course, are an essential part of many epidemiologic studies.

[1] Feinstein AR. *Clinimetrics*. New Haven and London: Yale University Press, 1987.

CLOSED COHORT A population in which membership begins at a defined time or with a defined event and ends only through occurrence of the study outcome or the end of eligibility for membership. An example is a population of women in labor being studied to determine the vital status of their offspring (i.e., whether live or stillborn).

CLUSTER Aggregation of relatively uncommon events or diseases in space and/or time in amounts that are believed or perceived to be greater than could be expected by chance.[1] Putative disease clusters are often perceived to exist on the basis of ANEC-

DOTAL EVIDENCE, and much effort may be expended by epidemiologists and biostatisticians in demonstrating whether a true cluster exists.

[1] National Conference on Clustering of Health Events. *Am J Epidemiol* 1990; 132:1 (Suppl) S1–S202.

CLUSTER ANALYSIS A set of statistical methods used to group variables or observations into strongly interrelated subgroups.

CLUSTERING (Syn: disease cluster, time cluster, time-place cluster) A closely grouped series of events or cases of a disease or other health-related phenomena with well-defined distribution patterns in relation to time or place or both. The term is normally used to describe aggregation of relatively uncommon events or diseases, e.g., leukemia, multiple sclerosis.

CLUSTER SAMPLING A sampling method in which each unit selected is a group of persons (all persons in a city block, a family, etc.) rather than an individual.

CODE A numerical and/or alphabetical system for classifying information, e.g., about diagnostic categories.

CODE OF CONDUCT A formal statement of desirable conduct that research workers and/or practitioners are expected to honor; there may be penalties for violation. Examples include the Hippocratic Oath, the Nürnberg (Nuremberg) Code, and the Helsinki Declaration, which govern requirements for research on human subjects. See also GUIDELINES.

CODING Translation of information, e.g., questionnaire responses, into numbered categories for entry in a data processing system.

COEFFICIENT OF CONCORDANCE A measure of the agreement among several rankings or categories.

COEFFICIENT OF VARIATION The ratio of the standard deviation to the mean. This is meaningful only if the variable is measured on a ratio scale. See MEASUREMENT SCALE.

COHERENCE The extent to which a hypothesized causal association is compatible with preexisting theory and knowledge.[1] Biological coherence requires compatibility with biological knowledge that may be derived from studies of nonhuman or human species.

[1] Susser MW. What is a cause and how do we know one? *Am J Epidemiol* 1991; 133:635–648.

COHORT (From Latin *cohors,* warriors, the tenth part of a legion)
1. The component of the population born during a particular period and identified by period of birth so that its characteristics (e.g., causes of death and numbers still living) can be ascertained as it enters successive time and age periods.
2. The term "cohort" has broadened to describe any designated group of persons who are followed or traced over a period of time, as in COHORT STUDY (prospective study).

COHORT ANALYSIS The tabulation and analysis of morbidity or mortality rates in relationship to the ages of a specific group of people (cohort) identified at a particular period of time and followed as they pass through different ages during part or all of their life span. In certain circumstances, e.g., studies of migrant populations, cohort analysis may be performed according to duration of residence of migrants in a country, rather than year of birth, in order to relate health or mortality experience to duration of exposure.

COHORT COMPONENT METHOD A method of population projection that takes the population distributed by age and sex at a base date and carries it forward in time on the basis of separate allowances for fertility, mortality, and migration.

COHORT EFFECT See GENERATION EFFECT.

COHORT INCIDENCE See INCIDENCE.

COHORT SLOPES Arrangement of data so that when plotted graphically, lines connect points representing the age-specific rates for population segments from the same generation of birth (see diagram). These slopes represent changes in rates with age during the life experience of each cohort.

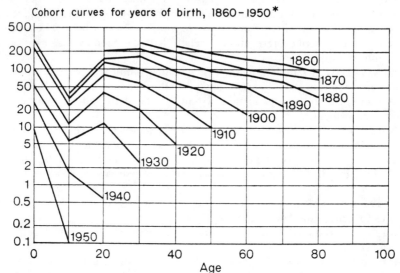

Cohort slopes. Tuberculosis mortality rates of successive birth generations; death rates for tuberculosis by age, United States, 1900–1960, per 100,000 population. From Susser, Watson, Hopper, 1985.

COHORT STUDY (Syn: concurrent, follow-up, incidence, longitudinal, prospective study) The analytic method of epidemiologic study in which subsets of a defined population can be identified who are, have been, or in the future may be exposed or not exposed, or exposed in different degrees, to a factor or factors hypothesized to influence the probability of occurrence of a given disease or other outcome. The main feature of cohort study is observation of large numbers over a long period (commonly years) with comparison of incidence rates in groups that differ in exposure levels. The alternative terms for a cohort study, i.e., follow-up, longitudinal, and prospective study, describe an essential feature of the method, which is observation of the population for a sufficient number of person-years to generate reliable incidence or mortality rates in the population subsets. This generally implies study of a large population, study for a prolonged period (years), or both.

COINTERVENTION In a RANDOMIZED CONTROLLED TRIAL, the application of additional diagnostic or therapeutic procedures to members of either or both the experimental and the control groups.

COLD CHAIN A system of protection against high environmental temperatures for heat-labile vaccines, sera, and other active biological preparations. Unless the cold chain is preserved, such preparations are inactivated and immunization procedures, etc., will be ineffective. Preservation of the cold chain is an integral part of the WHO expanded program on immunization in tropical countries.

COLLINEARITY Very high correlation between variables.

COLONIZATION See INFECTION.

COMMENSAL Literally, eating together (sharing the same table); an organism that lives harmlessly in the gut. See also XENOBIOTIC.

COMMON SOURCE EPIDEMIC (Syn: common vehicle epidemic) See EPIDEMIC, COMMON SOURCE.

COMMON VEHICLE SPREAD Transmission of a disease agent (infectious pathogen, toxic chemical, etc.) from a source that is common to those who acquire the disease. Common vehicles include air, water, food, injected substances. Legionellosis is an example of common vehicle spread in air that has passed through air conditioning equipment contaminated by the causal organism. HIV disease and hepatitis B and C can be spread among illicit drug users by the common vehicle of contaminated needles and syringes. Cholera and many other waterborne diseases are spread by the common vehicle of contaminated water. The principal modes of foodborne common vehicle spread were sonorously summarized by an anonymous author (probably Sir Andrew Balfour) in *Memoranda on Medical Diseases in Tropical and Subtropical Areas,*[1] published by the British War Office in 1914–1918, revised often in later wars: "careless carriers, contact cases, chiefly cooks, dirty drinking water, the dust of dried dejecta and the repulsive regurgitation, dangerous droppings, and filthy feet of faecal-feeding flies fouling food."

[1] London: HMSO, 1915, 1946, etc.

COMMUNICABLE DISEASE (Syn: infectious disease) An illness due to a specific infectious agent or its toxic products that arises through transmission of that agent or its products from an infected person, animal, or reservoir to a susceptible host, either directly or indirectly through an intermediate plant or animal host, vector, or the inanimate environment. See also TRANSMISSION OF INFECTION.

COMMUNICABLE PERIOD The time during which an infectious agent may be transferred directly or indirectly from an infected person to another person, from an infected animal to humans, or from an infected person to an animal, including arthropods. See also TRANSMISSION OF INFECTION.

COMMUNITY A group of individuals organized into a unit, or manifesting some unifying trait or common interest; loosely, the locality or catchment area population for which a service is provided, or more broadly, the state, nation, or body politic.

COMMUNITY DIAGNOSIS The process of appraising the health status of a community, including assembly of vital statistics and other health-related statistics and of information pertaining to determinants of health, such as prevalence of tobacco smoking, and examination of the relationships of these determinants to health in the specified community. The term may also denote the findings of this diagnostic process. Community diagnosis may attempt to be comprehensive or may be restricted to specific health conditions, determinants, or subgroups. J. N. Morris[1] identified community diagnosis as one of the uses of epidemiology.

[1] Morris JN: The uses of epidemiology. *Br Med J* 1955; 2:395–401.

COMMUNITY HEALTH See PUBLIC HEALTH.

COMMUNITY MEDICINE The study of health and disease in the population of a specified community. The goal is to identify health problems and needs, to identify means by which these needs may be met, and to evaluate the extent to which health services meet these needs. Also, the practice of medicine concerned with communities (or specified populations) rather than individuals; this includes the above elements and the organization and provision of health care at a community (or specified population) level.

COMMUNITY-ORIENTED PRIMARY HEALTH CARE Integration of community medicine with the primary health care of individuals.[1] The primary health care practitioner or team is responsible for health care both at the individual and at the community or population level.

[1] Institute of Medicine: *Community Oriented Primary Care*, Vols 1 and 2. Washington DC: National Academy Press, 1984.

See also PUBLIC HEALTH; SOCIAL MEDICINE.

COMMUNITY TRIAL Experiment in which the unit of allocation to receive a preventive or therapeutic regimen is an entire community or political subdivision. Examples include the trials of fluoridation of drinking water and of heart disease prevention in North Karelia (Finland) and California. See also CLINICAL TRIAL.

COMORBIDITY Disease(s) that coexist(s) in a study participant in addition to the index condition that is the subject of study.

COMPARISON GROUP Any group to which the index group is compared. Usually synonymous with control group.

COMPETING CAUSE When a previously common cause of death becomes rare, other causes become more prominent. These other causes are referred to as *competing causes*. For instance, among young adults, pneumonia and other infections were a common cause of death until about midway through the 20th century; their control has brought to prominence some competing causes of death, notably malignant disease and suicide.

COMPETING RISK An event that removes a subject from being at risk for the outcome under investigation. For example, in a study of smoking and cancer of the lung, a subject who dies of coronary heart disease is no longer at risk of lung cancer, and in this situation, coronary heart disease is a competing risk.

COMPLETED FERTILITY RATE The number of children born alive per woman in a cohort of women by the end of their childbearing years.

COMPLETING THE CLINICAL PICTURE The use of epidemiology to define all modes of presentation of a disease and/or all possible outcomes. One of the "uses of epidemiology" identified by J. N. Morris.[1]

[1] Morris JN: The use of epidemiology. *Br Med J* 2:395–401, 1955.

COMPLETION RATE The proportion or percentage of persons in a SURVEY for whom complete data are available for analysis. See also RESPONSE RATE.

COMPOSITE INDEX An index, such as the Apgar score, Tumor/Nodes/Metastates (TNM) stage of cancer, that contains contributions from categories of several different variables.

COMPRESSION OF MORBIDITY A term describing abbreviation of the average period of life when chronic illness or disability affects physical, mental, or social function. In theory, as health promotion and disease prevention become more efficacious, this period of long-term morbidity is compressed into a smaller proportion of the total life span. Empirical observations in several countries have failed to demonstrate the phenomenon. Others envisage an EXPANSION OF MORBIDITY or a state of balance. See also RECTANGULARIZATION OF MORTALITY.

COMPUTER A programmable electronic device that can be used to store and manipulate data in order to carry out designated functions. The two fundamental components of a computer are hardware, i.e., the actual electronic device, and software, the instructions or program used to carry out the function. Computer science has created a large language of its own, describing types of computers (main-frame, micro, digital, analogue, etc.) and all aspects of the process. Most of the terms used in this field are defined by A. J. Meadows, M. Gordon, and A. Singleton.[1]

[1] *Dictionary of New Information Technology.* London: Century, 1982.

COMPUTER VIRUS A self-replicating computer program capable of infecting other programs and spreading via data links to other computers, causing damage to or destruction of data files.

CONCORDANCE Pairs or groups of individuals of identical phenotype. In twin studies, a condition in which both twins exhibit or fail to exhibit a trait under investigation.

CONCORDANT A term used in TWIN STUDY to describe a twin pair in which both twins exhibit a certain trait.

CONCURRENT STUDY See COHORT STUDY.

CONDITIONAL PROBABILITY The probability of an event, given that another event has occurred. If D and E are two events and P (. . .) is "the probability of (. . .)," the conditional probability of D, given that E occurs, is denoted $P(D/E)$, where the vertical slash is read "given" and is equal to $P(D \text{ and } E)/P(E)$. The event E is the "conditioning event." Conditional probabilities obey all the axioms of probability theory. See also BAYES' THEOREM; PROBABILITY THEORY.

CONFIDENCE INTERVAL (CI) The computed interval with a given probability, e.g., 95%, that the true value of a variable such as a mean, proportion, or rate is contained within the interval.

CONFIDENCE LIMITS The upper and lower boundaries of the confidence interval.

CONFIDENTIALITY The obligation not to disclose information; the right of a person to withhold information from others. Information in medical records, case registries and other data files and bases is generally confidential, and epidemiologists are required to obtain permission before being given access to it; this may be the IN-FORMED CONSENT of the person to whom the records relate or the permission of an INSTITUTIONAL REVIEW BOARD. Epidemiologists have an obligation to preserve confidentiality of information they obtain during their studies. See also PRIVACY.

CONFLICT OF INTEREST Compromise of a person's objectivity when that person has a vested interest in peer review or outcome of a study; occurs when the person could benefit financially or in other ways (e.g., promotion, tenure) from some aspect of the study.

CONFOUNDING (From the Latin *confundere,* to mix together)
1. A situation in which the effects of two processes are not separated. The distortion of the apparent effect of an exposure on risk brought about by the association with other factors that can influence the outcome.
2. A relationship between the effects of two or more causal factors as observed in a set of data such that it is not logically possible to separate the contribution that any single causal factor has made to an effect.
3. A situation in which a measure of the effect of an exposure on risk is distorted because of the association of exposure with other factor(s) that influence the outcome under study.

CONFOUNDING VARIABLE, CONFOUNDER A variable that can cause or prevent the outcome of interest, is not an intermediate variable, and is associated with the factor under investigation. Unless it is possible to adjust for confounding variables, their effects cannot be distinguished from those of factor(s) being studied. Bias can occur when adjustment is made for any factor that is caused in part by the exposure and is also correlated with the outcome. For discussion, see Weinberg CR: Towards a clearer definition of confounding. *Am J Epidemiol* 1993;137:1–8.

CONSANGUINE Related by a common ancestor within the previous few generations.

CONSISTENCY

1. Close conformity between the findings in different samples, strata, or populations, or at different times or in different circumstances, or in studies conducted by different methods or different investigators. Consistency may be examined in order to study effect modification. Consistency of results on replication of studies is an important criterion in judgments of causality.

2. In statistics, an estimator is said to be consistent if the probability of its yielding estimates close to the true value approaches one as the sample size grows larger.

CONTACT (OF AN INFECTION) A person or animal that has been in such association with an infected person or animal or a contaminated environment as to have had opportunity to acquire the infection.

CONTACT, DIRECT A mode of transmission of infection between an infected host and susceptible host. Direct contact occurs when skin or mucous surfaces touch, as in shaking hands, kissing, and sexual intercourse. See also CONTAGION; TRANSMISSION OF INFECTION.

CONTACT, INDIRECT A mode of transmission of infection involving FOMITES or VECTORS. Vectors may be mechanical (e.g., filth flies) or biological (the disease agent undergoes part of its life cycle in the vector species). See also TRANSMISSION OF INFECTION.

CONTACT, PRIMARY Person(s) in direct contact or associated with a communicable disease case.

CONTACT, SECONDARY Person(s) in contact or associated with a primary contact.

CONTAGION The transmission of infection by direct contact, droplet spread, or contaminated FOMITES. These are the modes of transmission specified by Fracastorius (1484–1553) in *De Contagione* (1546); contemporary usage is sometimes looser, but use of this term is best restricted to description of infection transmitted by direct contact.

CONTAGIOUS Transmitted by contact; in common usage, "highly infectious."

CONTAINMENT The concept of regional eradication of communicable disease, first proposed by Soper in 1949 for the elimination of smallpox.[1] Containment of a worldwide communicable disease demands a globally coordinated effort so that countries that have effected an interruption of transmission do not become reinfected following importation from neighboring endemic areas.

[1] Pan American Health Organization, OSP, CE7, W-15, Washington DC, 1949.

CONTAMINATION

1. The presence of an infectious agent on a body surface; also on or in clothes, bedding, toys, surgical instruments or dressings, or other inanimate articles or substances including water, milk, and food. Pollution is distinct from contamination and implies the presence of offensive but not necessarily infectious matter in the environment. Contamination of a body surface does not imply a carrier state. See also TRANSMISSION OF INFECTION.

2. The situation that exists when a population being studied for one condition or factor also possesses other conditions or factors that modify results of the study. In a RANDOMIZED CONTROLLED TRIAL, the inadvertent application of the experimental procedure to members of the control group, or inadvertent failure to apply the procedure to members of the experimental group.

CONTINGENCY TABLE A tabular cross-classification of data such that subcategories of one characteristic are indicated horizontally (in rows) and subcategories of another characteristic are indicated vertically (in columns). Tests of association between the characteristics in the columns and rows can be readily applied. The simplest contingency table is the fourfold or 2×2 table. Contingency tables may be extended to include several dimensions of classification.

CONTINGENT VARIABLE See INTERMEDIATE VARIABLE.

CONTINUING SOURCE EPIDEMIC (OUTBREAK) An epidemic in which new cases of disease occur over a long period, indicating persistence of the disease source.

CONTINUOUS DATA, CONTINUOUS VARIABLE Data (variable) with a potentially infinite number of possible values along a continuum. Data representing a continuous variable include height, weight, and enzyme output.

CONTRACEPTIVE PREVALENCE RATE The percentage of married women of childbearing age who are using or whose husbands are using any form of contraception, whether modern or traditional. (Source: UNICEF.)

CONTROL

1. (v.) To regulate, restrain, correct, restore to normal.
2. (n. or adj.) Applied to many communicable and some noncommunicable conditions, *control* means ongoing operations or programs aimed at reducing the incidence and/or prevalence, or eliminating such conditions.
3. (n.) As used in the expressions *case control study* and *randomized control(led)* trial, *control* means person(s) in a comparison group that differs, respectively, in disease experience or allocation to a regimen from the subjects of the study.
4. (v.) In statistics, *control* means to adjust for or take into account extraneous influences or observations.
5. (adj.) In the expression *control variable*, we refer to an independent variable other than the hypothetical causal variable that has a potential effect on the dependent variable and is subject to control by analysis.

The use of the noun *control* to describe the comparison groups in a case control study and in a randomized control(led) trial can confuse the uninitiated, e.g., members of INSTITUTIONAL REVIEW BOARDS; the essential ethical distinction is that there may be no intervention in the lives or health status of the controls in a case control study, whereas controls in a randomized controlled trial may be asked to undergo a procedure or regimen that may affect their health; their informed consent is therefore essential. Consent may not be required (save to gain access to medical records) to study controls in a case control study. As Susser[1] has pointed out, the use of the word *control* as verb, adjective, and noun may confuse even careful readers. The verb is best used in the sense of controlling sources of extraneous variation in the dependent variable, whether by design or analysis. The verb is also used in the sense of controlling disease or its causes. The adjective is best used to describe control variables in contradistinction to uncontrolled and confounding variables. The adjective also can be used to describe a control group assembled for comparison with a group of cases or with an experimental group. The noun is best used to designate the members of a control group.

[1] *Causal Thinking in the Health Sciences.* New York: Oxford University Press, 1973.

CONTROL GROUP, CONTROLS Subjects with whom comparison is made in a case control study, randomized controlled trial, or other variety of epidemiologic study. Selection of appropriate controls is crucial to the validity of epidemiologic studies and has been much discussed.[1,2]

[1] Schlesselman JJ. *Case-Control Studies; Design, Conduct, Analysis.* New York: Oxford University Press, 1982.

[2] Wacholder S, McLaughlin JK, Silverman DT, Mandel JS: Selection of controls in case-control studies: I. Principles. *Am J Epidemiol* 1992; 135:1019–1028.

Wacholder S, Silverman DT, McLaughlin JK, Mandel JS. Selection of controls in case-control studies. II. Types of controls. *Am J Epidemiol* 1992; 135:1029–1041.

————: Selection of controls in case-control studies. III. Design options. *Am J Epidemiol* 1992; 135:1042–1050.

CONTROLS, HISTORICAL Persons or patients used for comparison who had the condition or treatment under study at a different time, generally at an earlier period than the study group or cases. Historical controls are often unsatisfactory because other factors affecting the condition under study may have changed to an unknown extent in the time elapsed.

CONTROLS, HOSPITAL Persons used for comparison who are drawn from the population of patients in a hospital. Hospital controls are often a source of SELECTION BIAS.

CONTROLS, MATCHED Controls who are selected so that they are similar to the study group, or cases, in specific characteristics. Some commonly used matching variables are age, sex, race, and socioeconomic status. See also MATCHING.

CONTROLS, NEIGHBORHOOD Persons used for comparison who live in the same locality as cases and therefore may resemble cases in environmental and socioeconomic criteria.

CONTROLS, SIBLING Persons used for comparison who are the siblings of cases and therefore share genetic makeup.

COORDINATES In a two-dimensional graph, the values of ordinate and abscissa that define the locus or position of a point.

CORDON SANITAIRE The barrier erected around a focus of infection. Used mainly in the isolation procedures applied to exclude cases and contacts of life-threatening communicable diseases from society. Mainly of historical interest.

CORRELATION The degree to which variables change together.

CORRELATION COEFFICIENT A measure of association that indicates the degree to which two variables have a linear relationship. This coefficient, represented by the letter r, can vary between $+1$ and -1; when $r = +1$, there is a perfect positive linear relationship in which one variable varies directly with the other; when $r = -1$, there is a perfect negative linear relationship between the variables. The measure can be generalized to quantify the degree of linear relationship between one variable and several others, in which case it is known as the multiple correlation coefficient. Kendall's Tau, Spearman's Rank Correlation, and Pearson's Product Moment Correlation tests are special varieties with occasional applications in epidemiology. Kendall and Buckland's *Dictionary of Statistical Terms*[1] gives details.

[1] London: Longman, 1983.

CORRELATION, NONSENSE A meaningless correlation between two variables. Nonsense correlations sometimes occur when social, economic, or technological changes have the same trend over time as incidence or mortality rates. An example is correlation between the birthrate and the density of storks in parts of Holland and Germany. See also CONFOUNDING; ECOLOGICAL FALLACY.

COST-BENEFIT ANALYSIS An economic analysis in which the costs of medical care and the benefits of reduced loss of net earnings due to preventing premature death or disability are considered. The general rule for the allocation of funds in a cost-benefit analysis is that the ratio of marginal benefit (the benefit of preventing an additional case) to marginal cost (the cost of preventing an additional case) should be equal to or greater than 1.

COST-EFFECTIVENESS ANALYSIS This form of analysis seeks to determine the costs and effectiveness of an activity or to compare similar alternative activities to determine the relative degree to which they will obtain the desired objectives or outcomes.

The preferred action or alternative is one that requires the least cost to produce a given level of effectiveness, or provides the greatest effectiveness for a given level of cost. In the health care field, outcomes are measured in terms of health status.

COST-UTILITY ANALYSIS A form of economic evaluation in which the outcomes of alternative procedures or programs are expressed in terms of a single "utility-based" unit of measurement. A widely used utility-based measure is the QUALITY-ADJUSTED LIFE YEAR.

COVARIATE A variable that is possibly predictive of the outcome under study. A covariate may be of direct interest to the study or may be a confounding variable or effect modifier.

COVERAGE A measure of the extent to which the services rendered cover the potential need for these services in a community. It is expressed as a proportion in which the numerator is the number of services rendered and the denominator is the number of instances in which the service should have been rendered. Example:

$$\frac{\text{Annual obstetric coverage}}{\text{in a community}} = \frac{\text{Number of deliveries attended by a qualified midwife or obstetrician}}{\text{Expected number of deliveries during the year in a given community}}$$

COX MODEL See PROPORTIONAL HAZARDS MODEL.

CRITERION A principle or standard by which something is judged. See also STANDARD.

CRITICAL APPRAISAL Application of rules of evidence to a study to assess the validity of the data, completeness of reporting, methods and procedures, conclusions, compliance with ethical standards, etc. The rules of evidence vary with circumstances. See also HIERARCHY OF EVIDENCE.

CRITICAL POPULATION SIZE The theoretical minimum host population size required to maintain an infectious agent. This size varies, depending on the agent and demographic, social, environmental conditions (hygiene, ambient temperature, etc), and, in the case of vector-borne diseases, the conditions required for survival and propagation of the vector species.

CRITICAL PERIOD, CRITICAL TIME WINDOW (Syn: etiologically relevant exposure period) The period during which exposure to a causal factor is relevant to causation of a disease.

CRONBACH'S ALPHA (Syn: internal consistency reliability) An estimate of the correlation between the total score across a series of items from a rating scale and the total score that would have been obtained had a comparable series of items been employed.

CROSS-CULTURAL STUDY A study in which populations from different cultural backgrounds are compared.

CROSS-DESIGN SYNTHESIS A method for evaluating outcomes of medical interventions developed by the US General Accounting Office (GAO). It is conducted by pooling databases such as the results of a RANDOMIZED CONTROLLED TRIAL (RCT) and of routinely treated patients, the latter database coming from hospital discharge statistics. Thus it is a variation of METAANALYSIS. This method is claimed to be more cost-effective than RCTs and more relevant to daily practice because it includes outcomes of patients in categories not included in RCTs; others assert that it is unreliable because some of the evidence comes from dubious sources. (Source: *Cross Design Synthesis: A New Strategy for Medical Effectiveness Research.* Washington, DC: General Accounting Office, 1992. See also *Lancet* 1992; 340:944–946.)

CROSS INFECTION Infection of one person with pathogenic organisms from another and vice versa. Not the same as NOSOCOMIAL INFECTION, which occurs in a health care setting; cross-infection can occur anywhere, e.g. in a military barracks, a school, a workplace.

CROSS-LEVEL BIAS A bias due to aggregation at the population level of causes and/or effects that are unlike at the individual level, occurring in ecologic studies. (For discussion, see Greenland S, Robins J. Ecologic studies—Biases, misconceptions and counter-examples. *Am J Epidemiol* 1994; 139:747–771.)

CROSSOVER DESIGN A method of comparing two or more treatments or interventions in which the subjects or patients, upon completion of the course of one treatment, are switched to another. In the case of two treatments, A and B, half the subjects are randomly allocated to receive these in the order A, B and half to receive them in the order B, A. A criticism of this design is that effects of the first treatment may carry over into the period when the second is given.

CROSS-PRODUCT RATIO See ODDS RATIO.

CROSS-SECTIONAL STUDY (Syn: disease frequency survey, prevalence study) A study that examines the relationship between diseases (or other health-related characteristics) and other variables of interest as they exist in a defined population at one particular time. The presence or absence of disease and the presence or absence of the other variables (or, if they are quantitative, their level) are determined in each member of the study population or in a representative sample at one particular time. The relationship between a variable and the disease can be examined (1) in terms of the prevalence of disease in different population subgroups defined according to the presence or absence (or level) of the variables and (2) in terms of the presence or absence (or level) of the variables in the diseased versus the nondiseased. Note that disease prevalence rather than incidence is normally recorded in a cross-sectional study. The temporal sequence of cause and effect cannot necessarily be determined in a cross-sectional study. See also MORBIDITY SURVEY.

CRUDE DEATH RATE See DEATH RATE.

CUMULATIVE DEATH RATE The proportion of a group that dies over a specified time interval. It may refer to all deaths or to deaths from specific cause(s). If follow-up is not complete on all persons, the proper estimation of this rate requires the use of methods that take account of CENSORING. Distinct from FORCE OF MORTALITY.

CUMULATIVE INCIDENCE, CUMULATIVE INCIDENCE RATE The number or proportion of a group of people who experience the onset of a health-related event during a specified time interval; this interval is generally the same for all members of the group, but, as in lifetime incidence, it may vary from person to person without reference to age.

CUMULATIVE INCIDENCE RATIO The ratio of the cumulative incidence rate in the exposed to the cumulative incidence rate in the unexposed.

CUSUM Acronym for cumulative sum (of a series of measurements). This is a useful way to demonstrate a change in trend or direction of a series of measurements.[1] Calculation begins with a reference figure, e.g., the expected average measurement. As each new measurement is observed, the reference figure is subtracted, and a cumulative total is produced by adding each successive difference. This cumulative total is the cusum.

[1] Alderson M: *An Introduction to Epidemiology*, 2nd ed. London: Macmillan, 1983.

CUT POINT An arbitrarily chosen point or value in an ordered sequence of values, used to separate the whole into parts. Commonly the cut point divides a distribution of values into parts that are arbitrarily designated as within or beyond the range considered normal. For example, a cut point of 85, 90, or 95 mm Hg differentiates normal from high blood pressure.

CYCLICITY, SEASONAL The annual cycling of incidence on a seasonal basis. Certain acute infectious diseases, if of greater than rare occurrence, peak in one season of the year and reach the low point 6 months later (or in the opposite season). The onset of some symptoms of some chronic diseases also may show this amplitudinal cyclicity. Demographic phenomena such as marriage and births, and mortality from all causes and certain specific causes, may also exhibit seasonal cyclicity.

CYCLICITY, SECULAR Fluctuation in disease incidence over a period longer than a year. For instance, in large, unimmunized populations, measles tends to have a 2-year cycle of high and low incidence. Empirical observations of secular and seasonal cycles of infectious diseases were the basis for epidemic theory, e.g., the MASS ACTION PRINCIPLE. Mass immunization programs, by raising herd immunity levels, have eliminated many such cycles.

CYST COUNT See WORM COUNT.

D

DALY See DISABILITY-ADJUSTED LIFE YEARS.

DATA A collection of items of information. Note: the singular of *data* is *datum;* in this age of sloppy speaking and writing, the plural noun is often accompanied by a singular verb.

DATABASE An organized set of data or collection of files that can be used for a specified purpose.

DATA CLEANING The process of excluding the information in incomplete, inconsistent records or irrelevant information collected in a survey or other form of epidemiologic study before analysis begins. This may mean excluding information that would distort the results if an attempt were made to edit and include it in the analysis, but it can also introduce biases. The fact that this step has been taken should be reported, along with the results of the study of analyzed data. See also RAW DATA.

DATA PROCESSING Conversion of items of information into a form that permits storage, retrieval, and analysis. Epidemiologic data may be transferred to punch cards, optical mark-sense cards, or directly into electronic files by computer. The term is loosely used to mean statistical analysis of data by means of a computer program.

DATA DREDGING A jargon term, meaning analyses done on a post hoc basis without benefit of prestated hypotheses, as a means of identifying noteworthy differences. Such analyses are sometimes done when data have been collected on a large number of variables and hypotheses are suggested by the data; the scientific validity of data dredging is at best dubious, usually unacceptable.

DEATH CERTIFICATE A vital record signed by a licensed physician or by another designated health worker that includes cause of death, decedent's name, sex, birth date, places of residence and of death, and whether the deceased had been medically attended before death. Occupation, birthplace, and other information may be included. Immediate cause of death is recorded on the first line, followed by conditions giving rise to the immediate cause; the underlying cause is entered last. The underlying cause is coded and tabulated in official publications of cause-specific mortality. Other significant conditions may also be recorded separately, as is the mode of death, whether accidental or violent, etc. The most important entries on a death certificate are underlying causes of death and cause of death. These are defined in the tenth (1990) revision of the INTERNATIONAL STATISTICAL CLASSIFICATION OF DISEASES AND RELATED HEALTH PROBLEMS (ICD-10) as follows:

Causes of death: The causes of death to be entered on the medical certificate of cause of death are all those diseases, morbid conditions, or injuries that either resulted in or contributed to death and the circumstances of the accident or violence which produced any such injuries.

Underlying cause of death: The underlying cause of death is (1) the disease or injury that initiated the train of events leading to death or (2) the circumstances of the accident or violence that produced the fatal injury.

Personal identifying information such as birthplace, parents' names (last name at birth), birth date, and personal identifying numbers are included on death certificates in some jurisdictions; this extra information makes possible a range of RECORD LINKAGE studies. See also INTERNATIONAL FORM OF MEDICAL CERTIFICATE OF CAUSES OF DEATH.

INTERNATIONAL FORM OF MEDICAL CERTIFICATE OF CAUSE OF DEATH

Cause of death		Approximate interval between onset and death
I Disease or condition directly leading to death*	(a) . . . . due to (or as a consequence of)	. . . .
Antecedent causes Morbid conditions, if any, giving rise to the above cause, stating the underlying condition last	(b) . . . . due to (or as a consequence of) (c) . . . . due to (or as a consequence of) (d)	. . . .
II Other significant conditions contributing to the death, but not related to the disease or condition causing it	. . . .	. . . .
*This does not mean the mode of dying, e.g. heart failure, respiratory failure. It means the disease, injury, or complication that caused death.		

Death certificate. The International Standard Form. From *International Statistical Classification of Diseases and Related Health Problems,* Tenth Revision (ICD-10) Vol. 2. Geneva: World Health Organization, 1991. With permission.

DEATH RATE An estimate of the proportion of a population that dies during a specified period. The numerator is the number of persons dying during the period; the denominator is the number in the population, usually estimated as the midyear population. The death rate in a population is generally calculated by the formula

$$\frac{\text{Number of deaths during a specified period}}{\text{Number of persons at risk of dying during the period}} \times 10^n$$

This rate is an estimate of the person-time death rate, i.e., the death rate per 10^n person-years. If the rate is low, it is also a good estimate of the cumulative death rate. This rate is also called the crude death rate.

DEATH REGISTRATION AREA A geographic area for which mortality data are collected, and, often, published.

DECISION ANALYSIS A derivative of OPERATIONS RESEARCH and GAME THEORY that involves identifying all available choices, and potential outcomes of each, in a series of decisions that have to be made about aspects of patient care—diagnostic procedures, therapeutic regimens, prognostic expectations. Epidemiologic data play a large part in determining the probabilities of outcomes following each choice that has to be made. The range of choices can be plotted on a DECISION TREE, and at each branch, or decision node, the probabilities of each outcome that can be predicted are displayed. The decision tree thus portrays the choices available to those responsible for patient care and the probabilities of each outcome that will follow the choice of a particular action or strategy in patient care. The relative worth of each outcome is preferably also described as a utility or quality of life, e.g., a probability of life expectancy or of freedom from disability,[1] often expressed as QALYs.

[1] Pauker SG, Kassirer JP. Decision analysis. *N Engl J Med* 1987; 316:250–258.

DECISION TREE The alternative choices expressed in quantitative terms, available at each stage in the process of thinking through a problem, may be likened to branches, and the hierarchical sequence of options to a tree. Hence, "decision tree." It is a graphic device used in DECISION ANALYSIS, in which a series of decision options are represented as branches and subsequent possible outcomes are represented as further branches. The decisions and the eventualities are presented in the order they are likely to occur. The junction where a decision must be taken is called a "decision node."

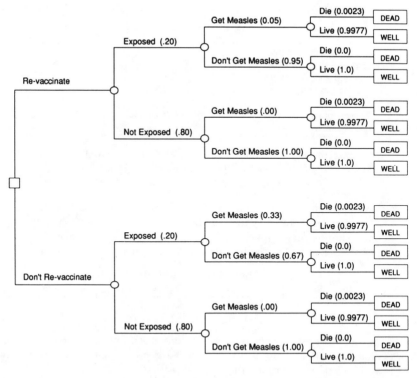

Decision tree. Probabilities of different outcomes with and without revaccination against measles. From Petitti DB: *Meta-Analysis, Decision Analysis and Cost-Effectiveness Analysis.* New York: Oxford University Press, 1994.

DEDUCTION Reasoned argument proceeding from the general to the particular.

DEGREES OF FREEDOM *(df)* The number of independent comparisons that can be made between the members of a sample. This important concept in statistical testing cannot be defined briefly. It refers to the number of independent contributions to a sampling distribution (such as χ^2, t, and F distribution). In a CONTINGENCY TABLE it is one less than the number of row categories multiplied by one less than the number of column categories.

DELPHI METHOD Iterative circulation to a panel of experts of questions and responses that are progressively refined in light of responses to each round of questions; preferably participants' identities should not be revealed to each other. The aim is to reduce the number of viable options or solutions, perhaps to arrive at a consensus judgment on an issue or problem, or a set of issues or problems, without allowing anyone to dominate the process. The method was developed at the RAND Corporation.

DEMAND (FOR HEALTH SERVICES) Willingness and/or ability to seek, use, and, in some settings, to pay for services. Sometimes further subdivided into *expressed demand* (equated with use) and *potential demand,* or *need.*

DEMOGRAPHIC TRANSITION The transition from high to low fertility (and mortality) rates in a country, formerly thought to be related to technologic change and industrialization but probably more directly related to female literacy and the status of women than to any other factors.

DEMOGRAPHIC TRAP The predicament of a population that has exceeded the CARRYING CAPACITY of its local or regional ecosystem and cannot afford to import food or other essentials:[1] people caught in the demographic trap become dependent upon external food aid, must emigrate as environmental refugees, or both. Another common outcome is conflict.[2]

[1] Population growth and ecological deterioration—the demographic trap, in *From Alma Ata to the Year 2000;* reflections at the mid-point. Geneva: WHO, 1988; pp 31–34.
[2] Last JM: War and the demographic trap. *Lancet* 1993, 342:508–509.

DEMOGRAPHY The study of populations, especially with reference to size and density, fertility, mortality, growth, age distribution, migration, and VITAL STATISTICS, and the interaction of all these with social and economic conditions.

DEMONSTRATION MODEL An experimental health care facility, program, or system with built-in provision for measuring aspects such as costs per unit of service, rates of use by patients or clients, and outcomes of encounters between providers and users. The aim usually is to determine the feasibility, efficacy, effectiveness, and/or efficiency of the model service.

DENOMINATOR The lower portion of a fraction used to calculate a rate or ratio. The population (or population experience, as in person-years, passenger-miles, etc.) at risk in the calculation of a rate or ratio. See also NUMERATOR.

DENSITY OF POPULATION Demographic term meaning numbers of persons in relation to available space.

DENSITY SAMPLING A method of selecting controls in a CASE CONTROL STUDY in which cases are sampled only from incident cases over a specific time period and controls are sampled and interviewed throughout that period (rather than simply at one point in time, such as the end of the period). This method can reduce bias due to changing exposure patterns in the source population.

DEPENDENCY RATIO Proportion of children and old people in a population in comparison to all others, i.e., the proportion of economically inactive to economically active; "children" are usually defined as ages under 15 and "old people" as ages 65 and over.

DEPENDENT VARIABLE

1. A variable the value of which is dependent on the effect of other variable(s)—independent variable(s)—in the relationship under study. A manifestation or outcome whose variation we seek to explain or account for by the influence of independent variables.
2. In statistics, the dependent variable is the one predicted by a regression equation.

See also INDEPENDENT VARIABLE.

DESCRIPTIVE STUDY A study concerned with and designed only to describe the existing distribution of variables, without regard to causal or other hypotheses. Contrast ANALYTIC STUDY. An example is a community health survey, used to determine the health status of the people in a community. Descriptive studies, e.g., analyses of cancer registry data, can be used to measure risks, generate hypotheses, etc.

DESIGN See RESEARCH DESIGN.

DESIGN BIAS The difference between a true value and that obtained as a result of faulty design of a study. Examples include uncontrolled studies where the effects of two or more processes cannot be separated (confounding); also studies done on poorly defined populations or with unsuitable control groups.

DESIGN EFFECT A BIAS in study findings attributable to the study design. A specific form is bias attributable to intraclass correlation in CLUSTER SAMPLING. The design effect for a cluster design is the ratio of the variance for that design to the variance calculated from a simple random sample of the same size.

DESIGN VARIABLE

1. A study variable whose distribution in the subjects is determined by the investigator.
2. In statistics, a variable taking on the value 1 to indicate membership in a particular category and 0 or −1 to indicate nonmembership in the category. Used primarily in ANALYSIS OF VARIANCE.

DESMOTERIC MEDICINE The practice of medicine in a prison. The infectious diseases of prisoners have become epidemiologically important since the onset of the HIV epidemic and proliferation of illicit intravenous drug use. The term was suggested by Tauxe and Patterson[1] and is derived from the Greek *desmoterion,* prison.

[1] Tauxe RB, Patterson CB: A word about prisons: "desmoteric." *N Engl J Med* 1988, 317:1669–1670.

DETECTION BIAS Bias due to systematic error(s) in methods of ascertainment, diagnosis, or verification of cases in an epidemiologic study. An example is verification of diagnosis by laboratory tests in hospital cases but failure to apply the same tests to cases outside the hospital.

DETERMINANT Any factor, whether event, characteristic, or other definable entity, that brings about change in a health condition or other defined characteristic. See also CAUSALITY.

DIAGNOSIS The process of determining health status and the factors responsible for producing it; may be applied to an individual, family, group, or community. The term is applied both to the process of determination and to its findings. See also DISEASE LABEL.

DIAGNOSIS-RELATED GROUP (DRG) Classification of hospital patients according to diagnosis and intensity of care required, used by insurance carriers to set reimbursement scales.

DIAGNOSTIC INDEX A system for recording diagnoses, diseases, or problems of patients or clients in a medical practice or service, usually including identifying information (name, birthdate, sex) and dates of encounters.

DIAGNOSTIC AND STATISTICAL MANUAL (DSM) A manual that aims to systematize and standardize the definitions of mental disorders developed by the American Psychiatric Association, listing all psychiatric diagnostic labels with the clinical and other criteria that can be used to establish the diagnosis. DSM-IV is the fourth edition, published in 1994.

DIFFERENTIAL The difference(s) shown in tabulation of health and vital statistics according to age, sex, or some other factor; age differentials are the differences revealed in the tabulations of rates in age groups, sex differentials are the differences in rates between males and females, income differentials are differences between designated income categories, etc.

DIGIT PREFERENCE A preference for certain numbers that leads to rounding off measurements. Rounding off may be to the nearest whole number, even number, multiple of 5 or 10, or (when time units like a week are involved) 7, 14, etc. This can be a form of OBSERVER VARIATION, or an attribute of respondent(s) in a survey.

DIMENSIONALITY The number of dimensions, i.e., scalar quantities, needed for accurate description of an element of a vector space.

DIRECT ADJUSTMENT, DIRECT STANDARDIZATION See STANDARDIZATION.

DIRECT OBSTETRICAL DEATH See MATERNAL MORTALITY.

DIRECTIONALITY

1. General term for the direction of inference of a study,[1] i.e., whether it is retrospective (backward-looking) or prospective (forward-looking).
2. The sign of a relationship between variables. Correlation coefficients are directional measures of association because the sign changes if one of the variables is reversed.

[1] Kramer MS, Boivin JF. Towards an "unconfounded" classification of epidemiologic research design. *J Chronic Dis* 1987; 40:683–688.

DIRECTIVES See GUIDELINES.

DISABILITY Temporary or long-term reduction of a person's capacity to function. See also INTERNATIONAL CLASSIFICATION OF IMPAIRMENTS, DISABILITIES, AND HANDICAPS for the official WHO definition.

DISABILITY-ADJUSTED LIFE YEARS (DALYS) A measure of the burden of disease on a defined population and the effectiveness of interventions. DALYs are advocated as an alternative to QALYs and claimed to be a valid indicator of population health.[1] They are based on adjustment of LIFE EXPECTANCY to allow for long-term disability as estimated from official statistics. However, their use as currently expressed and calculated may be limited because the necessary data are not available or do not exist. Moreover, the concept postulates a continuum from disease to disability to death that is not universally accepted, particularly by the community of persons with disabilities. See also DISABILITY-FREE LIFE EXPECTANCY.

[1] World Bank World Development Report 1993, *Investing in Health.*

DISABILITY-FREE LIFE EXPECTANCY (Syn: active life expectancy) The average number of years an individual is expected to live free of disability if current patterns of mortality and disability continue to apply.[1] A statistical abstraction based on existing age-specific death rates and either age-specific disability prevalences or age-specific disability transition rates.

[1] Mathers CD, Robine JM, Wilkins R: Health expectancy indicators; Recommendations for terminology, in Mathers CD, Robine JM, McCallum J, eds. *Proceedings of Seventh Meeting of the International Network on Health Expectancy (REVES).* Canberra: Aust Inst Health Welfare, 1994.

DISCORDANT A term used in TWIN STUDIES to describe a twin pair in which one twin exhibits a certain trait and the other does not. Also used in matched pair case control studies to describe a pair whose members had different exposures to the risk factor under study. Only the discordant pairs are informative about the association between exposure and disease.

DISCOUNT RATE A measure of costs, benefits, and outcomes in relation to time that allows for the fact that money (and health) have greater value in the present than at some future time. A term used mainly in economics and in CLINICAL DECISION ANALYSIS.

DISCRETE DATA Data that can be arranged into naturally occurring or arbitrarily selected groups or sets of values, as opposed to data in which there are no naturally occurring breaks in continuity, i.e., CONTINUOUS DATA. An example is number of decayed, missing, and filled teeth (DMF).

DISCRIMINANT ANALYSIS A statistical analytic technique used with discrete dependent variables, concerned with separating sets of observed values and allocating new values; can sometimes be used instead of regression analysis. Kendall and Buckland[1] refer to this as "discriminatory analysis" and describe it as a rule for allocating individuals or values from two or more discrete populations to the correct population with minimal probability of misclassification.

[1] Kendall MG, Buckland WR. *A Dictionary of Statistical Terms*, 4th ed. London: Longman, 1982.

DISEASE Literally, *dis-ease,* the opposite of *ease,* when something is wrong with a bodily function. The words *disease, illness,* and *sickness* are loosely interchangeable, but are better regarded as not synonymous. Susser[1] has suggested that they be used as follows:

Disease is a physiological/psychological dysfunction.

Illness is a subjective state of the person who feels aware of not being well;

Sickness is a state of social dysfunction, i.e., a role that the individual assumes when ill.

[1] Susser MW. *Causal Thinking in the Health Sciences.* New York: Oxford University Press, 1973.

DISEASE FREQUENCY SURVEY See CROSS-SECTIONAL STUDY; MORBIDITY SURVEY.

DISEASE LABEL The identity of the condition from which a patient suffers. It may be the name of a precisely defined disorder identified by a battery of tests, a probability statement based on consideration of what is most likely among several possibilities, or an opinion based on pattern recognition. Use of the word *label* can convey stigma, so this term should be used with care if at all. See also DIAGNOSIS.

DISEASE MAPPING A method for displaying spatial distribution of disease, most often used in veterinary epidemiology. Disease maps may display raw numbers or rates, i.e., CHOROPLETHIC MAPS.

DISEASE ODDS RATIO See ODDS RATIO.

DISEASE, PRECLINICAL Disease with no signs or symptoms because they have not yet developed. See also INAPPARENT INFECTION.

DISEASE REGISTRY See REGISTER, REGISTRY.

DISEASE, SUBCLINICAL A condition in which disease is detectable by special tests but does not reveal itself by signs or symptoms.

DISEASE TAXONOMY See TAXONOMY OF DISEASE.

DISINFECTION Killing of infectious agents outside the body by direct exposure to chemical or physical agents.

Concurrent disinfection is the application of disinfective measures as soon as possible after the discharge of infectious material from the body of an infected person, or after the soiling of articles with such infectious discharges, all personal contact with such discharges or articles being minimized prior to such disinfection.

Terminal disinfection is the application of disinfective measures after the patient has been removed by death or to a hospital, or has ceased to be a source of infection, or after other hospital isolation practices have been discontinued. Terminal disinfection is rarely practiced; terminal cleaning generally suffices, along with airing and sunning of rooms, furniture, and bedding. Disinfection is necessary only for diseases spread by indirect contact; steam sterilization or incineration of bedding and other items is desirable after a disease such as plague or anthrax.[1]

[1] Benenson AS, ed. *Control of Communicable Diseases in Man,* 15th ed. Washington DC: American Public Health Association 1990.

DISINFESTATION Any physical or chemical process serving to destroy or remove undesired small animal forms, particularly arthropods or rodents, present upon the person, the clothing, or in the environment of an individual, or on domestic animals. Disinfestation includes delousing for infestation with *Pediculus humanus humanus,* the body louse. Synonyms include the terms *disinsection* and *disinsectization* when insects only are involved.

DISTRIBUTION The complete summary of the frequencies of the values or categories of a measurement made on a group of persons. The distribution tells either how many or what proportion of the group was found to have each value (or each range of values) out of all the possible values that the quantitative measure can have.

DISTRIBUTION-FREE METHOD A method which does not depend upon the form of the underlying distribution.

DISTRIBUTION FUNCTION A function that gives the relative frequency with which a random variable falls at or below each of a series of values. Examples include the normal distribution, log-normal distribution, chi-square distribution, t distribution, F distribution, and binomial distribution, all of which have applications in epidemiology.

DMF The abbreviation DMF stands for decayed, missing, and filled teeth. Lowercase letters, i.e., dmf, are used for deciduous dentition, upper case for permanent teeth. The DMF number is widely used in dental epidemiology.

DOMINANT In genetics, alleles that fully manifest their phenotype when present in the heterozygous state. Contrast RECESSIVE.

DOSE-EFFECT RELATIONSHIP Association between dose (i.e., amount, duration, concentration) and magnitude of a graded effect in an individual or a population (cf. DOSE-RESPONSE RELATIONSHIP, which refers to a defined biological effect in an exposed population.) (After IUPAC Glossary.)

DOSE-RESPONSE RELATIONSHIP A relationship in which a change in amount, intensity, or duration of exposure is associated with a change—either an increase or a decrease—in risk of a specified outcome.

DOT CHART, DOT PLOT A display (plot) of the individual values of a set of numbers. The x axis represents categories of a noncontinuous variable, the y axis represents the values displayed by the observations.

DOUBLE-BLIND TRIAL A procedure of blind assignment to study and control groups and blind assessment of outcome, designed to ensure that ascertainment of outcome is not biased by knowledge of the group to which an individual was assigned. *Double* refers to both parties, i.e., the observer(s) in contact with the subjects and the subjects in the study and control groups. See also BLIND(ED) STUDY; RANDOMIZED CONTROLLED TRIAL.

DOUBLING TIME The average time taken for a population to double in numbers.

DRIFT See GENETIC DRIFT; SOCIAL DRIFT.

DROPLET NUCLEI A type of particle implicated in the spread of airborne infection. Droplet nuclei are tiny particles (1–10 μm diameter) that represent the dried residue of droplets. They may be formed by (1) evaporation of droplets coughed or

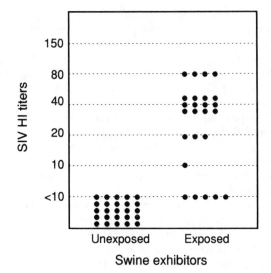

Dot chart, dot plot. Results of swine influenza virus (SIV) haemagglutination-inhibition (HI) antibody testing among exposed and unexposed swine exhibitors, Wisconsin, 1988. From Teutsch and Churchill, op. cit., 1994.

sneezed into the air or (2) aerosolization of infective materials. See also TRANSMISSION OF INFECTION.

DROPOUT A person enrolled in a study who becomes inaccessible or ineligible for follow-up, e.g., because of inability or unwillingness to remain enrolled in the study. The occurrence of dropouts can lead to biases in study results.

DUMMY VARIABLE See INDICATOR VARIABLE.

DYNAMIC POPULATION A population that gains and loses members; all natural populations are dynamic, a fact recognized by the term *population dynamics,* used by demographers to denote changing composition. See also POPULATION DYNAMICS; STABLE POPULATION.

E

e Symbol for the base of natural or Napierian logarithms, defined mathematically as the sum of the exponential series

$e^x = 1 + x + x^2/2! + x^3/3! + \ldots \ x^n/n!$ where $x = 1$ and n approaches infinity, i.e., $e = 1 + 1 + 1/2 + 1/6 + 1/24 + \ldots = 2.71828 \ldots$

EARLY WARNING SYSTEM In disease surveillance, a specific procedure to detect as early as possible any departure from usual or normally observed frequency of phenomena. For example, the routine monitoring of numbers of deaths from pneumonia and influenza in large American cities has been used as an early warning system for the identification of influenza epidemics. In developing countries, a change in children's average weights is an early warning signal of nutritional deficiency.

E-BOOK Method (developed by Eimerl)[1] of recording encounters in primary medical care: encounters are arranged by problem or diagnostic category, thus making it easy to count the number of persons seen (and the number of times each is seen) according to problem or diagnostic category in a given period of time. Widely used in epidemiologic studies of primary medical care. See also AGE-SEX REGISTER; DIAGNOSTIC INDEX.

[1] Eimerl TS: Organized curiosity. *J Coll Gen Pract* 3:246–252, 1960.

ECLOSION Emergence of imago (adult) from pupal case, hatching of larva from egg (descriptive of life stages of insect vectors).

ECOLOGICAL ANALYSIS Analysis based on aggregated or grouped data; errors in inference may result because associations may be artifactually created or masked by the aggregation process.

ECOLOGICAL CORRELATION A correlation in which the units studied are populations rather than individuals. Correlations found in this manner may not hold true for the individual members of these populations. See also ECOLOGICAL FALLACY.

ECOLOGICAL FALLACY (Syn: aggregation bias, ecological bias)
   1. The bias that may occur because an association observed between variables on an aggregate level does not necessarily represent the association that exists at an individual level.
   2. An error in inference due to failure to distinguish between different levels of organization.[1] A correlation between variables based on group (ecological) characteristics is not necessarily reproduced between variables based on individual characteristics; an association at one level may disappear at another, or even be reversed. Example: At the ecological level, a correlation has been found in several studies between the quality of drinking water and mortality rates from heart disease; it would be an ecological fallacy to infer from this

alone that exposure to water of a particular level of hardness necessarily influences the individual's chances of getting or dying of heart disease.

[1] Greenland S, Robins J: Ecologic studies—Biases, misconceptions and counter-examples. *Am J Epidemiol* 1994; 139:747–771.

ECOLOGICAL STUDY A study in which the units of analysis are populations or groups of people, rather than individuals. An example is the study of association between median income and cancer mortality rates in administrative jurisdictions such as states and counties.

ECOLOGY The study of the relationships among living organisms and their environment. *Human ecology* means the study of human groups as influenced by environmental factors, including social and behavioral factors.

ECOSYSTEM Plant and animal life considered in relation to the environmental factors that influence it; specifically, the fundamental unit in ecology, comprising the living organisms and the nonliving elements that interact in a defined region. This region may be any size, from a drop of pond water to the entire biosphere.

EFFECT The result of a cause. In epidemiology, frequently a synonym for EFFECT MEASURE.

EFFECTIVENESS In the usage made standard among epidemiologists by A. L. Cochrane (1909–1988), effectiveness is a measure of the extent to which a specific intervention, procedure, regimen, or service, when deployed in the field in routine circumstances, does what it is intended to do for a specified population.[1] To be distinguished from EFFICACY and EFFICIENCY.

[1] Cochrane AL. *Effectiveness and Efficiency; Random Reflections on Health Services.* London: Nuffield Provincial Hospitals Trust, 1972.

EFFECT MEASURE A quantity that measures the effect of a factor on the frequency or risk of a health outcome. Three such measures are attributable fractions, which measure the fraction of cases due to a factor; risk and rate differences, which measure the amount a factor adds to the risk or rate of a disease; and risk and rate ratios, which measure the amount by which a factor multiplies the risk or rate of disease.

EFFECT MODIFIER (Syn: conditional variable, moderator variable) A factor that modifies the effect of a putative causal factor under study. For example, age is an effect modifier for many conditions, and immunization status is an effect modifier for the consequences of exposure to pathogenic organisms. Effect modification is detected by varying the selected effect measure for the factor under study across levels of another factor. See also CAUSALITY, FACTORS IN; INTERACTION.

EFFECTIVE POPULATION SIZE The average number of individuals in a population that contribute genes to the next generation.

EFFECTIVE SAMPLE SIZE Sample size after dropouts, deaths, and other specified exclusions from an original sample.

EFFICACY The extent to which a specific intervention, procedure, regimen, or service produces a beneficial result under ideal conditions. Ideally, the determination of efficacy is based on the results of a RANDOMIZED CONTROLLED TRIAL.

EFFICIENCY

1. The effects or end results achieved in relation to the effort expended in terms of money, resources, and time. The extent to which the resources used to provide a specific intervention, procedure, regimen, or service of known efficacy and effectiveness are minimized. A measure of the economy (or cost in resources) with which a procedure of known efficacy and effectiveness is carried out.

2. In statistics, the relative precision with which a particular study design or estimator will estimate a parameter of interest.

EGG COUNT See WORM COUNT.

ELIGIBILITY CRITERIA An explicit statement of the conditions under which persons are admitted to an epidemiologic study, e.g., a case control study or a randomized controlled trial.

ELIMINATION Reduction of case transmission to a predetermined very low level; e.g., elimination of tuberculosis as a public health problem was defined by the WHO (1991) as reduction of prevalence to a level below one case per million population. Compare ERADICATION (OF DISEASE).

E-MAIL See INFORMATION SUPERHIGHWAY.

EMERGING PATHOGENS This term describes a general class of infectious organisms that have recently come to the attention of clinicians, infectious disease specialists, and epidemiologists. Several, such as the human immunodeficiency virus, *Borrelia burgdorferi* (responsible for Lyme disease), and hantaviruses have well-defined epidemiologic features. Epidemiologic studies can undoubtedly clarify causes and suggest control measures for many such pathogens, whether they are indeed "new" i.e., newly evolved organisms, or "old" i.e., organisms that have long existed but have only lately been discovered to be capable of infecting humans.

EMPIRICAL Based directly on experience, e.g., observation or experiment, rather than on reasoning alone.

EMPORIATRICS The specialty of travel medicine. The term first appeared in J. E. Banta's "Treating the traveler; a brief guide to emporiatrics." (*Postgrad Med J* 1973; 53:7:53–58). The word comes from the Greek *emporion* (trade); it is most commonly used by writers on tropical diseases.

ENCOUNTER A face-to-face transaction between a personal health worker and a patient or client.

ENDEMIC DISEASE The constant presence of a disease or infectious agent within a given geographic area or population group; may also refer to the usual prevalence of a given disease within such area or group. See also HOLOENDEMIC DISEASE; HYPERENDEMIC DISEASE.

ENDOBIOTIC An endogenous substance that is metabolized with adverse effects, such as development of cancer. Contrast XENOBIOTIC.

END RESULTS See OUTCOMES.

ENVIRONMENT All that which is external to the individual human host. Can be divided into physical, biological, social, cultural, etc., any or all of which can influence health status of populations.

ENVIRONMENTAL EPIDEMIOLOGY Study of the effect on human health of physical, chemical, and biological factors in the external environment.[1]

[1] *Environmental Epidemiology.* Washington, DC: National Research Council, Vol 1, 1991; Vol 2, 1995.

ENVIRONMENTAL HEALTH CRITERIA DOCUMENT Official publication containing a review of existing knowledge about chemicals, radiation, etc., and their identifiable immediate and long-term effects on health. Environmental health criteria documents are produced by the WHO, the International Agency for Research on Cancer (IARC), and many national agencies, such as the National Institute for Occupational Safety and Health (NIOSH) in the USA.

ENVIRONMENTAL HEALTH IMPACT ASSESSMENT A statement of the beneficial or adverse health effects or risks due to an environmental exposure or likely to follow an environmental change. Such statements may contain or refer to results of epidemiologic and/or toxicologic studies of environmental health hazards.

ENVIRONMENTAL HYPERSENSITIVITY An ill-defined, perhaps nonexistent condition, attributed to exposure to very small amounts of chemical and other agents encountered in urban settings.

ENVIRONMENTAL TOBACCO SMOKE (ETS) A specific form of air pollution due to burning tobacco, especially sidestream smoke. ETS is a confirmed carcinogen.[1]

[1] Environmental Protection Agency: *Respiratory Health Effects of Passive Smoking: Lung Cancer and Other Disorders.* Washington DC: Office of Health and Environmental Assessment, 1992.

EPIDEMIC [from the Greek *epi* (upon), *dēmos* (people)] The occurrence in a community or region of cases of an illness, specific health-related behavior, or other health-related events clearly in excess of normal expectancy. The community or region and the period in which the cases occur are specified precisely. The number of cases indicating the presence of an epidemic varies according to the agent, size, and type of population exposed; previous experience or lack of exposure to the disease; and time and place of occurrence. Epidemicity is thus relative to usual frequency of the disease in the same area, among the specified population, at the same season of the year. A single case of a communicable disease long absent from a population or first invasion by a disease not previously recognized in that area requires immediate reporting and full field investigation; two cases of such a disease associated in time and place may be sufficient evidence to be considered an epidemic. Recent epidemics initially identified following the occurrence of small numbers of cases include the epidemic of vaginal cancer in daughters of women who took diethylstilbestrol during pregnancy[1] and the pandemic of AIDS that was heralded by a report[2] of cases of *Pneumocystis carinii* pneumonia among gay men in Los Angeles in 1981. The purpose of surveillance systems such as the EPIDEMIC INTELLIGENCE SERVICE is to identify epidemics as early as possible so that effective control measures can be put in place. This remains the most important use for epidemiology.

The word may be used also to describe outbreaks of disease in animal or plant populations. See also EPIZOOTIC; EPORNITHIC.

[1] Herbst AL, Ulfelder H, Poskanzer DC. Adenocarcinoma of the vagina: Association of maternal stilbestrol therapy with tumor appearance in young women. *N Engl J Med* 1971; 284:878–881.

[2] Centers for Disease Control: Pneumocystic pneumonia—Los Angeles. *MMWR* 1981; 30:250–252.

EPIDEMIC, COMMON SOURCE (Syn: common vehicle epidemic, holomiantic disease) Outbreak due to exposure of a group of persons to a noxious influence that is common to the individuals in the group. When the exposure is brief and essentially simultaneous, the resultant cases all develop within one incubation period of the disease (a "point" or "point source" epidemic).

The term *holomiantic disease* was used by Stallybrass (1931) to describe outbreaks of this type, but as with several other terms created from Greek or Latin roots, transmission to epidemiologists who lacked a classical education did not take place.

EPIDEMIC CURVE A graphic plotting of the distribution of cases by time of onset.

EPIDEMIC INTELLIGENCE SERVICE (EIS) A training and service program developed in 1951 in the US Public Health Service Communicable Diseases Center (now the Centers for Disease Control and Prevention) by Alexander Langmuir (1910–1993) to investigate epidemics with unusual features: large or life-threatening epidemics, outbreaks of previously unidentified conditions, etc. As of 1994, the program has trained over 2000 EIS officers. Similar services modeled on the EIS have been developed in other countries.

EPIDEMIC, MATHEMATICAL MODEL OF See MATHEMATICAL MODEL.

EPIDEMICS, HISTORY OF The effect of diseases on the course of history fascinates epidemiologists and historians alike. It has preoccupied scholars since the biblical plagues, Hippocrates, and the epidemic, described by Thucydides, that struck the Athenians at the end of the first year of the Peloponnesian War (429 B.C.). Measles and smallpox brought by Europeans defeated the Aztecs and Incas, who in return gave tobacco and perhaps syphilis to Europeans. There are innumerable scholarly and popular works on the subject. Early treatises include those of Hecker[1] and Creighton[2]; a modern work by a historian is *Plagues and Peoples.*[3] Perhaps the nearest to a comprehensive monograph by an epidemiologist is Thomas McKeown's *The Origins of Human Disease.*[4] Partial accounts include histories of the impact on societies and civilizations of syphilis,[5] tuberculosis,[6] poliomyelitis,[7] typhus[8] and many other conditions.[9]

[1] Hecker JFK. *Der grossen Volkskrankheiten des Mittelalters* (Epidemics of the Middle Ages). Berlin: Enslin, 1865 (English translation published by the Sydenham Society, London, 1883).
[2] Creighton C. *A History of Epidemics in Britain.* Cambridge: Cambridge University Press, 1891–1994 (2 Vols).
[3] New York: Doubleday, 1976.
[4] Oxford: Blackwell, 1988.
[5] Pusey WA. *The History and Epidemiology of Syphilis.* Springfield, IL: Thomas, 1933.
[6] Dubos R, Dubos J. *The White Plague; Tuberculosis, Man and Society.* Boston: Little, Brown, 1952.
[7] Paul JR: *A History of Poliomyelitis.* New Haven, CT: Yale University Press, 1971.
[8] Zinsser H: *Rats, Lice and History.* Boston: Little, Brown, 1935.
[9] Grmek MD: *Les Maladies à L'Aube de la Civilization Occidentale.* Paris: Payot, 1983.

EPIDEMIC, POINT SOURCE See EPIDEMIC, COMMON SOURCE.

EPIDEMIC THRESHOLD The number or density of susceptibles required for an epidemic to occur. According to the MASS ACTION PRINCIPLE, the epidemic threshold is the reciprocal of the INFECTION TRANSMISSION PARAMETER.

EPIDEMIOLOGIC TRANSITION THEORY According to Omran,[1] the mortality component of the DEMOGRAPHIC TRANSITION has well defined phases: (1) The "age of pestilence and famine;" (2) the "age of receding pandemics;" (3) the "age of degenerative and man-made diseases." Omran says the shift from the first to third phases took about 100 years in the western industrial nations, but occurred more rapidly in Japan and Eastern Europe; many developing countries have yet to undergo the shift. Mackenbach[2] asserts that the transition from first to third phase took considerably longer in western industrial nations; and that "degenerative and man-made diseases" is a misleading term for conditions such as cancer and cardiovascular disease, which have complex etiologies.

[1] Omran AR: The epidemiologic transition; a theory of the epidemiology of population change. *Milbank Mem Fund Quart,* 1971, 49:509–538.
[2] Mackenbach JP: The epidemiologic transition theory. *J Epidemiol Community Health* 1994, 48:329–332.

EPIDEMIOLOGIST An investigator who studies the occurrence of disease or other health-related conditions or events in defined populations. The control of disease in populations is often also considered to be a task for the epidemiologist, especially in speaking of certain specialized fields such as malaria epidemiology. Epidemiologists may study disease in populations of animals and plants, as well as among human populations. See also CLINICAL EPIDEMIOLOGIST.

EPIDEMIOLOGY The study of the distribution and determinants of health-related states or events in specified populations, and the application of this study to control of health problems. "Study" includes surveillance, observation, hypothesis testing, analytic research, and experiments. "Distribution" refers to analysis by time, place, and classes of persons affected. "Determinants" are all the physical, biological, social, cultural, and behavioral factors that influence health. "Health-related states and events" include diseases, causes of death, behavior such as use of tobacco, reactions to preventive regimens, and provision and use of health services. "Specified populations" are those with identifiable characteristics such as precisely defined numbers. "Application to control . . ." makes explicit the aim of epidemiology—to promote, protect, and restore health.

There have been many definitions of epidemiology. In the past 50 years or so, the definition has broadened from concern with communicable disease epidemics to take in all phenomena related to health in populations.

The *Oxford English Dictionary (OED)* gives as a definition: "That branch of medical science which treats of epidemics" and cites Parkin (1873) as a source. However, there was a "London Epidemiological Society" in the 1850s. The identity of the scholar who first used the word at that time has been lost. *Epidemiologia* appears in the title of a Spanish history of epidemics, *Epidemiologia española,* Madrid, 1802.

Epidemic is much older. The word appears in Johnson's *Dictionary* (1775), and *OED* gives a citation dated 1603. The word was, of course, used by Hippocrates.

EPIDEMIOLOGY, ANALYTIC See ANALYTIC STUDY.

EPIDEMIOLOGY, DESCRIPTIVE Study of the occurrence of disease or other health-related characteristics in human populations. General observations concerning the relationship of disease to basic characteristics such as age, sex, race, occupation, and social class; also concerned with geographic location. The major characteristics in descriptive epidemiology can be classified under the headings: persons, place, and time. See also OBSERVATIONAL STUDY.

EPIDEMIOLOGY, EXPERIMENTAL See EXPERIMENTAL EPIDEMIOLOGY.

EPISODE Period in which a health problem or illness exists, from its onset to its resolution. See also ENCOUNTER.

EPIZOOTIC An outbreak (epidemic) of disease in an animal population (often with the implication that it may also affect human populations).

EPORNITHIC An outbreak (epidemic) of disease in a bird population.

EQUIPOISE A state of genuine uncertainty about the benefits or harms that may result from each of two or more regimens. A state of equipoise is an indication for a RANDOMIZED CONTROLLED TRIAL, because there are no ethical concerns about one regimen being better for a particular patient.

ERADICATION (OF DISEASE) Termination of all transmission of infection by extermination of the infectious agent through surveillance and containment. Eradication, as in the instance of smallpox, was based on the joint activities of control and surveillance. Regional eradication has been successful with malaria and in some countries appears close to succeeding for measles. The term *elimination* is sometimes used to describe eradication of diseases such as measles from a large geographic region or political jurisdiction. In 1992, the WHO put it this way: Eradication is defined as achievement of a status whereby no further cases of a disease occur anywhere, and continued control measures are unnecessary. Smallpox was eradicated in 1977, an eradication based on joint control and surveillance activities. Current candidates for eradication are poliomyelitis and dracunculosis.[1]

See also ELIMINATION.

[1] *WHO Weekly Epidemiological Record* 1990; 65:48:369–376.

ERROR

1. A false or mistaken result obtained in a study or experiment. Several kinds of error can occur in epidemiology, for example, due to bias.
2. Random error is the portion of variation in a measurement that has no appar-

ent connection to any other measurement or variable, generally regarded as due to chance.

3. Systematic error, which often has a recognizable source, e.g., a faulty measuring instrument, or pattern, i.e., it is consistently wrong in a particular direction. See also BIAS.

ERROR, TYPE I (Syn: alpha error) The error of rejecting a true null hypothesis i.e., declaring that a difference exists when it does not. See also SIGNIFICANCE; STATISTICAL TEST.

ERROR, TYPE II (Syn: beta error) The error of failing to reject a false null hypothesis i.e., declaring that a difference does not exist when in fact it does. See also POWER; STATISTICAL TEST.

ESTIMATE A measurement or a statement about the value of some quantity is said to be an estimate if it is known, believed, or suspected to incorporate some degree of error.

ESTIMATOR In statistics, a function for computing estimates of a parameter from observed data.

ETHICS The branch of philosophy that deals with distinctions between right and wrong—with the moral consequences of human actions. Ethical principles govern the conduct of epidemiology, as they do all human activities. The ethical issues that arise in epidemiologic practice and research include informed consent, confidentiality, respect for human rights, and scientific integrity. Epidemiologists and others have developed guidelines for the ethical conduct of epidemiologic studies.[1,2]

[1] Bankowski Z, Bryant JH, Last JM, eds. *Ethics and Epidemiology: International Guidelines.* Geneva: CIOMS/WHO, 1991.

[2] Fayerweather WE, Higginson J, Beauchamp TL, eds. *Ethics in Epidemiology.* New York: Pergamon Press, 1991 (also *J Clin Epidemiol* 1991; 44, suppl I).

ETHICS (ETHICAL) REVIEW COMMITTEE See INSTITUTIONAL REVIEW BOARD.

ETHNIC GROUP A social group characterized by a distinctive social and cultural tradition, maintained within the group from generation to generation, a common history and origin, and a sense of identification with the group. Members of the group have distinctive features in their way of life, shared experiences and often a common genetic heritage. These features may be reflected in their health and disease experience. See also RACE.

ETIOLOGIC FRACTION (EXPOSED) See ATTRIBUTABLE FRACTION (EXPOSED).

ETIOLOGIC FRACTION (POPULATION) See ATTRIBUTABLE FRACTION (POPULATION).

ETIOLOGY Literally, the science of causes, causality; in common usage, cause. See also CAUSALITY; PATHOGENESIS.

EVALUATION A process that attempts to determine as systematically and objectively as possible the relevance, effectiveness, and impact of activities in the light of their objectives. Several varieties of evaluation can be distinguished, e.g., evaluation of structure, process, and outcome. See also CLINICAL TRIAL; EFFECTIVENESS; EFFICACY; EFFICIENCY; HEALTH SERVICES RESEARCH; PROGRAM EVALUATION AND REVIEW TECHNIQUES; QUALITY OF CARE.

EVANS'S POSTULATES Expanding biomedical knowledge has led to revision of the HENLE–KOCH POSTULATES. Alfred Evans[1] developed those that follow, based on the Henle-Koch model.

1. Prevalence of the disease should be significantly higher in those exposed to the hypothesized cause than in controls not so exposed.
2. Exposure to the hypothesized cause should be more frequent among those

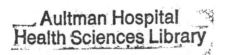

with the disease than in controls without the disease—when all other risk factors are held constant.

3. Incidence of the disease should be significantly higher in those exposed to the hypothesized cause than in those not so exposed, as shown by prospective studies.

4. The disease should follow exposure to the hypothesized causative agent with a normal or log-normal distribution of incubation periods.

5. A spectrum of host responses should follow exposure to the hypothesized agent along a logical biological gradient from mild to severe.

6. A measurable host response following exposure to the hypothesized cause should have a high probability of appearing in those lacking this before exposure (e.g., antibody, cancer cells) or should increase in magnitude if present before exposure. This response pattern should occur infrequently in persons not so exposed.

7. Experimental reproduction of the disease should occur more frequently in animals or humans appropriately exposed to the hypothesized cause than in those not so exposed; this exposure may be deliberate in volunteers, experimentally induced in the laboratory, or may represent a regulation of natural exposure.

8. Elimination or modification of the hypothesized cause should decrease the incidence of the disease (i.e., attenuation of a virus, removal of tar from cigarettes).

9. Prevention or modification of the host's response on exposure to the hypothesized cause should decrease or eliminate the disease (i.e., immunization, drugs to lower cholesterol, specific lymphocyte transfer factor in cancer).

10. All of the relationships and findings should make biological and epidemiologic sense.

[1] Evans AS: Causation and disease: The Henle-Koch postulates revisited. *Yale J Biol Med* 1976; 49:175–195.

EVIDENCE-BASED MEDICINE The process of finding relevant information in the medical literature to address a specific clinical problem; the application of simple rules of science and common sense to determine the validity of the information; the application of the information to the clinical question. In short, patient care based on evidence derived from the best available ("gold standard") studies. See CRITICAL APPRAISAL, HIERARCHY OF EVIDENCE.

EXACT METHOD A statistical method based on the actual, i.e., "exact" probability distribution of the study data, rather than on an approximation such as the normal or chi-square distribution; for example, Fisher's exact test.

EXACT TEST A statistical test based on the actual null probability distribution of the study data, rather than, say, normal approximation. The most common exact test is the Fisher-Irwin test for fourfold tables.

EXCESS RATE AMONG EXPOSED See RATE DIFFERENCE.

EXCESS RISK A term sometimes used to refer to the POPULATION EXCESS RATE and sometimes to RISK DIFFERENCE.

EXPANDED PROGRAMME ON IMMUNIZATION Part of the effort to achieve "Health for All by the Year 2000," under the auspices of WHO, UNICEF, and other international and bilateral aid agencies. This is a program of immunizing against diphtheria, tetanus, measles, pertussis, poliomyelitis, and tuberculosis, conducted especially in developing countries.

EXPANSION OF MORBIDITY As life expectancy increases, the prevalence of long-term disease, especially among older persons, increases. Mental disorders such as dementia may be an example.[1] Thus this is the opposite of COMPRESSION OF MORBIDITY. Both phenomena may co-exist in the same population, some disorders becoming less prevalent, others more so.

[1] Kramer JM. The rising pandemic of mental disorders and associated chronic diseases and disabilities. *Acta Psychiatr Scand* 1980; 62 (suppl 285):382–397.

EXPECTATION OF LIFE (Syn: life expectancy or expectation) The average number of years an individual of a given age is expected to live if current mortality rates continue to apply. A statistical abstraction based on existing age-specific death rates.

Life expectancy at birth ($\mathring{e}_0$): Average number of years a newborn baby can be expected to live if current mortality trends continue. Corresponds to the total number of years a given birth cohort can be expected to live, divided by the number of children in the cohort. Life expectancy at birth is partly dependent on mortality in the first year of life; therefore it is lower in poor than in rich countries because of the higher infant and child mortality rates in the former.

Life expectancy at a given age, age x ($\mathring{e}_x$): The average number of additional years a person age x would live if current mortality trends continue to apply, based on the age-specific death rates for a given year.

Life expectancy is a hypothetical measure and indicator of current health and mortality conditions. It is not a rate.

EXPERIMENT A study in which the investigator intentionally alters one or more factors under controlled conditions in order to study the effects of so doing.

EXPERIMENTAL EPIDEMIOLOGY In modern usage, this term is often equated with RANDOMIZED CONTROLLED TRIALS. To epidemiologists in the 1920s, it meant the study of epidemics among colonies of experimental animals such as rats and mice. The original meaning of the term is preferable; if the word *experiment* is qualified by the adjective *epidemiologic,* it is a synonym for RANDOMIZED CONTROLLED TRIAL. Clinical or community-based studies only merit the term *experiment* or *quasi-experiment* if it is possible to modify conditions during the period of study. See also ANIMAL MODEL.

EXPERIMENTAL STUDY A study in which conditions are under the direct control of the investigator. In epidemiology, a study in which a population is selected for a planned trial of a regimen whose effects are measured by comparing the outcome of the regimen in the experimental group with the outcome of another regimen in a control group. To avoid BIAS members of the experimental and control groups should be comparable except in the regimen that is offered them. Allocation of individuals to experimental or control groups is ideally by randomization. In a RANDOMIZED CONTROLLED TRIAL, individuals are randomly allocated; in some experiments, e.g., fluoridation of drinking water, whole communities have been (nonrandomly) allocated to experimental and control groups.

EXPLANATORY STUDY A study whose main objective is to explain, rather than merely describe, a situation by isolating the effects of specific variables and understanding the mechanisms of action. See also PRAGMATIC STUDY.

EXPLANATORY VARIABLE
1. A variable that causally explains the association or outcome under study.
2. In statistics, a synonym for INDEPENDENT VARIABLE.

EXPOSED In epidemiology, the exposed group (or simply, *the exposed*) is often used to connote a group whose members have been exposed to a supposed cause of a disease or health state of interest or possess a characteristic that is a determinant of the health outcome of interest.

EXPOSURE

1. Proximity and/or contact with a source of a disease agent in such a manner that effective transmission of the agent or harmful effects of the agent may occur.
2. The amount of a factor to which a group or individual was exposed; sometimes contrasted with dose, the amount that enters or interacts with the organism.
3. Exposures may of course be beneficial rather than harmful, e.g., exposure to immunizing agents.

EXPOSURE ASSESSMENT Process of estimating concentration or intensity, duration and frequency of exposure to an agent that can affect health. (Based on IUPAC Glossary.)

EXPOSURE CONTROL See HAZARD IDENTIFICATION.

EXPOSURE LIMIT General term defining the regulated level of exposure that should not be exceeded. (Based on IUPAC Glossary.)

EXPOSURE-ODDS RATIO See ODDS RATIO.

EXPOSURE RATIO The ratio of rates at which persons in the case and control groups of a CASE CONTROL STUDY are exposed to the RISK FACTOR (or to the protective factor) of interest.

EXPRESSIVITY In genetics, the extent to which a gene is expressed.

EXTRAPOLATE, EXTRAPOLATION To predict the value of a variate outside the range of observations; the resulting prediction. See also INTERPOLATE.

EXTREMAL QUOTIENT The ratio of the rate in the geographic region with the highest rate of interventions such as surgical procedures to the rate in the region with the lowest rate.[1]

[1] Kazandjian VA. The extremal quotient as a measure of variation in the rate of surgical procedures. *Health Serv Res* 1989; 24:665–684. [there aren't any "et al's"]

EXTRINSIC INCUBATION PERIOD Time required for development of a disease agent in a vector from the time of uptake of the agent to the time when the vector is infective. See also INCUBATION PERIOD; VECTOR-BORNE INFECTION.

F

F DISTRIBUTION (Syn: variance ratio distribution) The distribution of the ratio of two independent quantities each of which is distributed like a variance in normally distributed samples. So named in honor of R. A. Fisher (1890–1962), who first described this distribution.

F_1 ("F one") Term used in genetics to describe first-generation progeny of a mating.

FACTOR (Syn: determinant)

1. An event, characteristic, or other definable entity that brings about a change in a health condition or other defined outcome. See also CAUSALITY, CAUSATION OF DISEASE, FACTORS IN.

2. A synonym for (categorical) independent variable, or more precisely, an independent variable used to identify, with numerical codes, membership of qualitatively different groups. A causal role may be implied, as in "overcrowding is a factor in disease transmission," where overcrowding represents the highest level of the factor "crowding."

FACTOR ANALYSIS A set of statistical methods for analyzing the correlations among several variables in order to estimate the number of fundamental dimensions that underlie the observed data and to describe and measure those dimensions. Used frequently in the development of scoring systems for rating scales and questionnaires.

FACTORIAL DESIGN A method of setting up an experiment or study to assure that all levels of each intervention or classificatory factor occur with all levels of the others.

FALSE NEGATIVE Negative test result in a subject who possesses the attribute for which the test is conducted. The labeling of a diseased person as healthy when screening in the detection of disease. See also SCREENING; SENSITIVITY AND SPECIFICITY.

FALSE POSITIVE Positive test result in a subject who does not possess the attribute for which the test is conducted. The labeling of a healthy person as diseased when screening in the detection of disease. See also SCREENING; SENSITIVITY AND SPECIFICITY.

FAMILIAL DISEASE Disease that exhibits a tendency to familial occurrence. Familial occurrence of disease may be due to genetic transmission, intrafamilial transmission of infection or culture, interaction within the family, or the family's shared experience, including its exposure to a common environment.

FAMILY A group of two or more persons united by blood, adoptive or marital ties, or the common-law equivalent; the family may include members who do not share the household but are united to other members by blood, adoptive or marital, or equivalent ties. Epidemiologic studies may be concerned with family members or with those who share the same household or dwelling unit.

FAMILY, EXTENDED A group of persons comprising members of several generations united by blood, adoptive and marital, or equivalent ties. See also FAMILY, NUCLEAR.

FAMILY CONTACT DISEASE Disease that occurs among members of the family of a worker who is exposed to a toxic substance such as asbestos dust and carries this home on his person or his clothing, causing exposure to other family members.

FAMILY, NUCLEAR A group of persons comprising members of a single or at most two generations, usually husband-wife-children, united by blood or adoptive and marital or equivalent ties.

FAMILY OF CLASSIFICATIONS The Conference for the Tenth Revision of the International Statistical Classification of Diseases and Related Health Problems recommended adopting the concept of the family of disease and health-related classifications.[1] This "family" comprises ICD-10 (the ICD three-character core classification), its short tabulation lists, and the ICD four-character classification; lay reporting and other community based information schemes in health; specialty-based adaptations for oncology, psychiatry, etc.; other health-related classifications (ICIDH, procedures, reasons for encounter); and the International Nomenclature of Diseases (IND).

Family of disease and health-related classifications

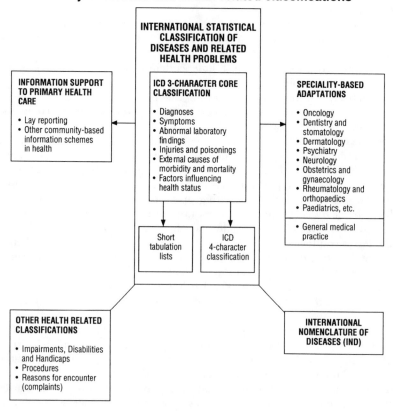

The WHO Family of Classifications. From *International Statistical Classification of Diseases and Related Health Problems,* Tenth Revision (ICD-10) Vol. 1. Geneva: World Health Organization, 1991. With permission.

[1] *ICD-10,* Vol 1: Report of the International Conference for the Tenth Revision of the International Classification of Diseases (pp. 9–28, Vol 1, ICD-10). Geneva: WHO, 1993.

FAMILY STUDY An epidemiologic study of a family or a group of families. The term has been used to describe surveillance of family groups, e.g., for tuberculosis. In genetics, investigation of families showing an unusual characteristic in order to determine whether the characteristic clusters in certain families, and if so, why.

FARR'S LAWS OF EPIDEMICS William Farr (1807–1883), who was the first Compiler of Abstracts in the General Register Office of England and Wales, enunciated several "laws" of epidemics.[1] He defined the relationship of incidence and prevalence. He observed that epidemics appear to be generated in unhealthy places, go through a regular course, and decline. In his Second Annual Report (1840) he demonstrated mathematically that the decline in mortality of a waning epidemic occurs at a uniformly accelerating rate. He constructed mathematical models to explain the natural history of epidemic diseases, often correctly and elegantly.

[1] Farr W. *Vital Statistics; A Memorial Volume of Selections from the Reports and Writings of William Farr.* Edited by Noel Humphries. London: Stanford, 1885.

FATALITY RATE The death rate observed in a designated series of persons affected by a simultaneous event, e.g., victims of a disaster. A term to be avoided, because it can be confused with CASE FATALITY RATE.

FEASIBILITY STUDY Preliminary study to determine practicability of a proposed health program or procedure, or of a larger study, and to appraise the factors that may influence its practicability. See also PILOT INVESTIGATION STUDY.

FECUNDITY The ability to produce live offspring. Fecundity is difficult to measure since it refers to the theoretical ability of a woman to conceive and carry a fetus to term. If a woman produces a live birth, it is known that she and her consort were fecund during some time in the past.

FEMALE-MALE GAP A set of national, regional, or other estimates—for example, of health status, literacy—in which all the figures for females are expressed as a percentage of the corresponding figures for males, which are indexed to 100. (Source: UNICEF.)

FERTILITY The actual production of live offspring. Stillbirths, fetal deaths, and abortions are not included in the measurement of fertility in a population. See also GRAVIDITY; PARITY.

FERTILITY RATE See GENERAL FERTILITY RATE.

FERTILITY RATIO A measure of the fertility of the population that restricts the denominator to the female population of appropriate age for childbearing. The fertility ratio is defined as

$$\text{Fertility ratio} = \frac{\text{Number of girls under 15 years of age}}{\text{Number of women in 15–49 age group}} \times 1000$$

(Not to be confused with GENERAL FERTILITY RATE.)

FETAL DEATH (Syn: stillbirth) Death prior to the complete expulsion or extraction from its mother of a product of conception, irrespective of the duration of pregnancy. The death is indicated by the fact that after such separation the fetus does not breathe or show any other evidence of life, such as beating of the heart, pulsation of the umbilical cord, or definite movement of voluntary muscles. Defined variously as death after the 20th or 28th week of gestation (the definition of the length of gestation varies between different jurisdictions, making this event difficult to compare internationally). The WHO Conference for the Tenth Revision of the International Classification of Diseases (ICD-10) recommended that the definition of fetal death should remain unchanged. See also LIVE BIRTH.

FETAL DEATH CERTIFICATE (Syn: certificate of stillbirth) A vital record registering a fetal death or stillbirth. Some health jurisdictions require the use of a fetal death certificate for all products of conception, whereas others require its use only in cases in which gestation has reached a particular duration, usually the 20th or the 28th week.

FETAL DEATH RATE (Syn: stillbirth rate) The number of fetal deaths in a year expressed as a proportion of the total number of births (live births plus fetal deaths) in the same year.

$$\text{Fetal death rate} = \frac{\text{Number of fetal deaths in a year}}{\begin{array}{c}\text{Number of fetal deaths plus live}\\\text{births in the same year}\end{array}} \times 1000$$

Note that the denominator is larger than for the FETAL DEATH RATIO and that the fetal death rate is therefore lower than the fetal death ratio, which is used in some jurisdictions. International comparisons of stillbirth or fetal death statistics will be flawed if the distinction is not appreciated.

FETAL DEATH RATIO A measure of fetal wastage, related to the number of live births. Defined as

$$\text{Fetal death ratio} = \frac{\text{Number of fetal deaths in a year}}{\text{Number of live births in the same year}}$$

(Can be expressed as a rate per 1000.)

FIELD SURVEY The planned collection of data in "the field," i.e., usually among non-institutionalized persons in the general population. A method of establishing a relationship between two or more variables in a population in numerical terms by eliciting and collating information from existing sources (not only records but people who can say how they feel or what happened). See also CROSS-SECTIONAL STUDY.

FISHER'S EXACT TEST The test for association in a two-by-two table that is based upon the exact hypergeometric distribution of the frequencies within the table.

FISHING EXPEDITION Exploratory study to find clues and leads for further study. Although the term is sometimes used pejoratively, "fishing expeditions" may be done for worthwhile causes, e.g., to seek clues to the cause of a major life-threatening outbreak. A recent example was the initial investigation of Legionnaires' disease.

FITNESS This word has specific meanings in several fields related to epidemiology.
1. In population genetics, a measure of the relative survival and reproductive success of a given phenotype or population subgroup.
2. In health promotion, health risk appraisal, physical fitness is a set of attributes that people have or achieve that relate to their ability to perform physical activity. Intellectual and emotional fitness can also be described and to some extent measured.

FIXED COHORT A cohort in which membership is fixed by being present at some defining event ("zero time"); an example is the cohort comprising survivors of the atomic bomb exploded at Hiroshima. See also CLOSED COHORT.

FLOW DIAGRAM (Syn: Logic model) A diagram comprising blocks connected by arrows representing steps in a process. An ALGORITHM used in decision analysis. Flow diagrams have many uses, e.g., to show eligibility, recruitment, and losses in design and execution of a study.

FOCUS OF INFECTION As used in malaria epidemiology, a defined and circumscribed locality containing the epidemiologic factors needed for transmission: a human community, a source of infection, a vector population, and appropriate environmental conditions. The term can be applied to other infectious diseases.

FOLLOW-UP Observation over a period of time of an individual, group, or initially defined population whose appropriate characteristics have been assessed in order to observe changes in health status or health-related variables. See also COHORT.

FOLLOW-UP STUDY
1. A study in which individuals or populations, selected on the basis of whether they have been exposed to risk, received a specified preventive or therapeutic procedure, or possess a certain characteristic, are followed to assess the outcome of exposure, the procedure, or effect of the characteristic, e.g., occurrence of disease.
2. Synonym for COHORT STUDY.

FOMITES (singular, fomes) Articles that convey infection to others because they have been contaminated by pathogenic organisms. Examples include handkerchief, drinking glass, door handle, clothing, and toys.

FORCE OF MORBIDITY (Syn: hazard rate, instantaneous incidence density, instantaneous incidence rate, person-time incidence rate) Theoretical measure of the number of new cases that occur per unit of population-time, e.g., person-years at risk. This is a measure of the occurrence of disease at a point in time, t, defined mathematically as the limit, as Δt approaches zero, of

$$\frac{\text{Probability that a person well at time } t \text{ will develop the disease in the interval } t+\Delta t}{\Delta t}$$

The average value of this quantity over the interval t to $(t+\Delta t)$ can be estimated as

$$\frac{\text{Incident cases observed from } t \text{ to } (t+\Delta t)}{\text{Number of person-time units of experience observed from } t \text{ to } (t+\Delta t)}$$

FORCE OF MORTALITY (Syn: actuarial death rate) The hazard rate of the occurrence of death at a point in time t, i.e., the limit as Δt approaches zero, of the probability that an individual alive at time t will die by time $t+\Delta t$, divided by Δt. Distinct from cumulative death rate.

FORECASTING A method of estimating what may happen in the future that relies on extrapolation of existing trends (demographic, epidemiologic, etc.). It may be less useful than SCENARIO BUILDING, which has greater flexibility. For example, extrapolation of mortality trends for coronary heart disease in the early 1960s in the United States suggested that the mortality rates would continue to rise, whereas in fact the rates began to fall soon after that time.

FORTUITOUS RELATIONSHIP A relationship that occurs by chance and needs no further explanation.

FORWARD SURVIVAL ESTIMATE A procedure for estimating the age distribution at some later date by projecting forward an observed age distribution. The procedure uses survival ratios, often obtained from model life tables.

FOURFOLD TABLE See CONTINGENCY TABLE.

"FOURTH WORLD" The environmental and socioeconomic situation of decayed urban neighborhoods in affluent nations, resembling the conditions encountered in the poorest developing countries. Homeless people are among an underclass (often disenfranchised) found in urban communities in rich countries. This term should not be used without explanation in scientific writing; it is included here because it is not found in standard dictionaries.

FRACTALS Mathematical patterns developed by Benoit Mandelbrot in 1977, in which small parts have the same shape as the whole. Blood vessels and the bronchial tree behave according to fractal theory. An application of fractals is in studies of the way human and other populations grow and spread. The same rules may apply to the spread of some infections and neoplasms.

FRAGILE DATA Data derived from a well-designed study that do not quite reach a level of statistical significance but arrive at unexpected and/or important conclusions. Alternatively, data that reach or imply important conclusions from a poorly designed study. A term preferably avoided.

FOURFOLD TABLE See CONTINGENCY TABLE.

FRAMINGHAM STUDY Probably the best known cohort study of heart disease. Since 1949, samples of residents of Framingham, Massachusetts, have been subjects of investigations of risk factors in relation to the occurrence of heart disease and later, other outcomes.

FREQUENCY See OCCURRENCE.

FREQUENCY DISTRIBUTION See DISTRIBUTION.

FREQUENCY MATCHING See MATCHING.

FREQUENCY POLYGON A graphic illustration of a distribution, made by joining a set of points, for each of which the abscissa is the midpoint of the class and the ordinate, or height, is the frequency.

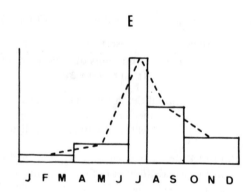

Frequency polygon. Numbers of notified cases in specified months. From Abramson JH, *Making Sense of Data*, 2nd Ed. 1994.

FUNCTION A quality, trait, or fact that is so related to another as to be dependent upon and to vary with this other.

FUNNEL PLOT A plotting device used in METAANALYSIS to detect PUBLICATION BIAS. The estimate of risk is plotted against sample size.[1] If there is no publication bias, the plot is funnel-shaped; but if studies showing significant results are more likely to be published, there is a "hole in the lower left corner" of the funnel.

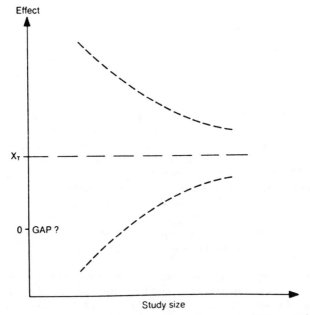

Funnel plot. From Dickerson and Berlin, op. cit. With permission.

[1] Dickerson K, Berlin JA. Meta-analysis: State of the science. *Epidemiol Rev* 1992; 14:154–176.

G

GAUSSIAN DISTRIBUTION See NORMAL DISTRIBUTION.

GAME THEORY A branch of mathematical logic developed by von Neumann and Morgenstern[1] concerned with the range of possible reactions to a particular strategy; each reaction can be assigned a probability and each reaction can lead to further action by the "adversary" in the game. Used mainly in systems analysis and such applications as war-gaming, game theory has occasional applications in disease surveillance and control. It is also one of the underlying theories used in clinical decision analysis.

[1] von Neumann J, Morgenstern O. *Theory of Games and Economic Theory.* New York: Wiley, 1947.

GATEKEEPER A person or system that selectively regulates or controls access to a health care service.

GAY (Since circa 1970, n, adj) Homosexual. The devastating impact of HIV disease on members of the gay community in several large cities prompted epidemiologic studies that clarified many details of the natural history of AIDS and have led to effective health education aimed at control of the epidemic.

GENDER In grammar, the term to designate a noun (person, animal, or object) as masculine, feminine or neuter. In parts of the English-speaking world, *gender* now signifies the totality of culturally determined awareness, attitudes, and beliefs about males and females and sometimes their sexual orientation. This usage may be politically correct, or a form of what Fowler[1] calls genteelism. When *gender* replaces the semantically correct word, sex—for instance, in the headings of statistical tables—it is bewildering to readers whose first language has nouns that may carry any of three genders that are not necessarily related to the sex of the individual (e.g., German: *das Mädchen,* the girl).

[1] Fowler HW. *Modern English Usage,* 2nd Ed., Revised and edited by Sir Ernest Gowers. Oxford and New York: Oxford University Press 1965.

GENE A sequence of DNA that codes for a particular protein product or that regulates other genes. Genes are the biological basis of heredity and occupy precisely defined locations on chromosomes.

GENE POOL The total of all genes possessed by reproductive members of a population.

GENERAL FERTILITY RATE A more refined measure of fertility than the crude birthrate. The denominator is restricted to the number of women of childbearing age (i.e., 15–44 or 15–49. Defined as

$$\text{General fertility rate} = \frac{\text{Number of live births in an area during a year}}{\text{Midyear female population age 15–44 in same area in same year}} \times 1000$$

The upper age limit for this rate is 44 years in most jurisdictions.

GENERATION EFFECT (Syn: cohort effect) Variation in health status that arises from the different causal factors to which each birth cohort in the population is exposed as the environment and society change. Each consecutive birth cohort is exposed to a unique environment that coincides with its life span.

GENERATION TIME The interval between receipt of infection by and maximal infectivity of the host. This applies to both clinical cases and inapparent infections.

With person-to-person transmission of infection, the interval between cases is determined by the generation time. See SERIAL INTERVAL. See also INCUBATION PERIOD.

GENETIC DRIFT Random variation in gene frequency from generation to generation; most often observed in small populations. The process of evolution through random statistical fluctuation of genetic composition of populations.

GENETIC ENGINEERING Manipulation of genome of a living organism.

GENETIC EPIDEMIOLOGY The science that deals with the etiology, distribution and control of disease in groups of relatives, and with inherited causes of disease in populations. The study of the role of genetic factors and their interaction with environmental factors in the occurrence of disease in human populations. This study has made rapid progress since the development of MOLECULAR EPIDEMIOLOGY.

GENETIC LINKAGE Particular genes occupy specific sites in chromosomes, one member of each pair of chromosomes of course coming from each parent. When two genes are fairly close to each other in the same chromosome pair, they tend to be inherited together. Such genes are said to be linked, and the phenomenon is called genetic linkage.

GENETIC PENETRANCE The extent to which a genetically determined condition is expressed in an individual. This determines the frequency with which genetic effect is shown in a population.

GENETICS The branch of biology dealing with heredity and variation of individual members of a species. Its branches include population genetics, which overlaps epidemiology; therefore we include pertinent genetic terms in this dictionary.

GENOME The array of genes carried by an individual.

GEOGRAPHIC PATHOLOGY (Syn: medical geography) The comparative study of countries, or of regions within them, with regard to variations in morbidity/mortality. The (implied) aim of such study is usually to demonstrate that the variations are caused by or related to differences in the geographic environment.

GEOMETRIC MEAN See MEAN, GEOMETRIC.

GESTATIONAL AGE Strictly speaking, the gestational age of a fetus is the elapsed time since conception. However, as the moment when conception occurred is rarely known precisely, the duration of gestation is measured from the first day of the last normal menstrual period. Gestational age is expressed in completed days or completed weeks (e.g., events occurring 280–286 days after the onset of the last normal menstrual period are considered to have occurred at 40 weeks of gestation).

Measurements of fetal growth, as they represent continuous variables, are expressed in relation to a specific week of gestational age (e.g., the mean birth weight for 40 weeks is that obtained at 280–286 days of gestation on a weight-for-gestational-age curve). Some specified variations of gestational age are: *Preterm:* Less than 37 completed weeks (less than 259 days). *Term:* From 37 to less than 42 completed weeks (259–293 days). *Postterm:* Forty-two completed weeks or more (294 days or more).

GLOBAL BURDEN OF DISEASE Indicator of the loss of healthy life years from disease, measured in DISABILITY-ADJUSTED LIFE YEARS. (Source: World Bank: *World Development Report*, 1993.)

GLOVER PHENOMENON Variation, apparently haphazard, in rates at which common procedures such as tonsillectomy are conducted in seemingly comparable communities with comparable morbidity rates; probably due to varying therapeutic fashions.[1]

[1]Glover JA. The incidence of tonsillectomy in school children. *Proc R Soc Med* 1938; 31:1219–1236.

GOAL A desired state to be achieved within a specified time. See also TARGET.

"GOLD STANDARD" (jargon) A method, procedure, or measurement that is widely accepted as being the best available. Often used to compare with new methods.

GOMPERTZ-MAKEHAM FORMULA A formula describing the relationship of mortality rate to age. There is an age-independent component and a component that increases exponentially with age. Benjamin Gompertz, a 19th-century demographer, first identified the proportionate relationship of mortality to age. This was refined by W. M. Makeham in 1867 to provide a better model of the age-specific pattern of the instantaneous death rate. If q_x is the probability of dying at age x and A, B, and C are constants, $q_x = A + BC^x$. For ages beyond childhood, the Gompertz-Makeham formula closely fits observed patterns.

GONADOTROPHIC CYCLE One complete round of ovarian development in the mosquito (or other insect vector) from the time when the blood meal is taken to the time when the fully developed eggs are laid.

GOODNESS OF FIT Degree of agreement between an empirically observed distribution and a mathematical or theoretical distribution.

GOODNESS-OF-FIT TEST A statistical test of the hypothesis that data have been randomly sampled or generated from a population that follows a particular theoretical distribution or model. The most common such tests are chi-square tests.

GRADIENT OF INFECTION The variety of host responses to infection ranging from inapparent infection to fatal illness.

GRAPH Visual display of the relationship between variables; the values of one set of variables are plotted along the horizontal or x axis, of a second variable, along the

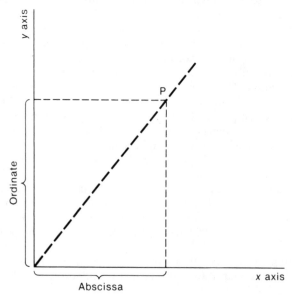

Graph showing abscissa, ordinate and locus of a point, P, in relation to x and y axis.

vertical or *y* axis. Three-dimensional graphs of relationships between three variables can be represented and comprehended visually in two dimensions. The relationship between *x* and *y* may be linear, exponential, logarithmic, etc. See also AXIS, ABSCISSA, ORDINATE. "Graph" is also a descriptive term for histograms, bar charts, etc.

GRAVIDITY The number of pregnancies (completed or incomplete) experienced by a woman.

"GRAY LITERATURE" (Syn: fugitive literature) Reports that are unpublished, have limited distribution, and are not included in bibliographic retrieval systems. Such reports may come from local or regional health departments or unpublished masters' or doctoral dissertations. Gray literature, including epidemiologic studies, although not usually peer-reviewed, may contain useful scientific findings, including information that might occasionally be useful in METAANALYSIS.

GROSS REPRODUCTION RATE The average number of female children a woman would have if she survived to the end of her childbearing years and if, throughout that period, she were subject to a given set of age-specific fertility rates and a given sex ratio at birth. This rate provides a measure of replacement fertility in the absence of mortality. See also NET REPRODUCTION RATE.

GROWTH RATE OF POPULATION A measure of population growth (in the absence of migration) comprising addition of newborns to the population and subtraction of deaths. The result, known as *natural rate of increase,* is calculated as

$$\frac{\text{Live births during the year } - \text{ deaths during the year}}{\text{Midyear population}} \times 1000$$

Alternatively, it is the difference between crude birthrate and crude death rate.

GUIDELINES A formal statement about a defined task or function. Examples include clinical practice guidelines, guidelines for application of preventive screening procedures, and guidelines for ethical conduct of epidemiologic practice and research.[1] Contrast CODE OF CONDUCT, in which the rules are intended to be strictly adhered to and may include penalties for violation. In the terminology developed by the European Community, *directives* are stronger than *recommendations,* which are stronger than *guidelines.* In North America, *guidelines* is normal usage also for recommendations.

[1] McDonald CJ, Overhage JM: Guidelines you can follow and can trust: An ideal and an example. *JAMA* 1994; 271:872–873.

GUTTMAN SCALE A measurement scale that ranks response categories to a question, with each unit representing an increasingly strong expression of an attribute such as pain, disability, or an attitude.

H

HACKETT SPLEEN CLASSIFICATION A numerical means of recording the size of an enlarged spleen, especially in malaria. This is a 6-point scale of 0 (no enlargement) to 5 (enlarged to umbilicus or larger). See *Terminology of Malaria and of Malaria Eradication.* Geneva: WHO, 1963:40–41.

HALF-LIFE Time in which the concentration of a substance is reduced by 50%.

HALO EFFECT

1. The effect (usually beneficial) that the manner, attention, and caring of a provider have on a patient during a medical encounter regardless of what medical procedures or services the encounter involves. See also PLACEBO, PLACEBO EFFECT.
2. The influence upon an observation of the observer's perception of the characteristics of the individual observed (other than the characteristic under study) or the influence of the observer's recollection or knowledge of findings on a previous occasion.

HANDICAP Reduction in a person's capacity to fulfill a social role as a consequence of an IMPAIRMENT, inadequate training for the role, or other circumstances. Applied to children, the term usually refers to the presence of an impairment or other circumstance that is likely to interfere with normal growth and development or with the capacity to learn. See also INTERNATIONAL CLASSIFICATION OF IMPAIRMENTS, DISABILITIES, AND HANDICAPS for the official WHO definition.

HANDICAP-FREE LIFE EXPECTANCY The average number of years an individual is expected to live free of handicap if current patterns of mortality and handicap continue to apply.[1] See also DISABILITY-FREE LIFE EXPECTANCY, HEALTH EXPECTANCY.

[1] Mathers CD, Robine JM, Wilkins R. Health expectancy indicators; Recommendations for terminology, in Mathers CD, Robine JM, McCallum J, eds. *Proceedings of Seventh Meeting of the International Network on Health Expectancy (REVES).* Canberra: Australian Institute of Health and Welfare, 1994.

HAPHAZARD SAMPLE Selection of a group for study without thought as to whether they are representative of the population. The word *haphazard* here implies selection based on a mixture of criteria such as convenience, accessibility, turning up at the time an investigation or study is in progress, and belonging to some existing list or registry, etc. Because they have an unknown chance of being unrepresentative of the population, haphazard samples are unsatisfactory for generalization.

HARDY-WEINBERG LAW The principle that both gene and genotype frequencies will remain in equilibrium in an infinitely large population in the absence of mutation, migration, selection, and nonrandom mating. If p is the frequency of one allele and q is the frequency of another and $p+q=1$, then p^2 is the frequency of homozygotes for the allele, q^2 is the frequency of homozygotes for the other allele, and $2pq$ is the frequency of heterozygotes.

HARMONIC MEAN See MEAN, HARMONIC.

HAWTHORNE EFFECT The effect (usually positive or beneficial) of being under study upon the persons being studied; their knowledge of the study often influences their behavior. The name derives from work studies by Whitehead, Dickson, Roethlisberger, and others, in the Western Electric Plant, Hawthorne, Illinois, reported by Elton Mayo in *The Social Problems of an Industrial Civilization* (London: Routledge, 1949).

HAZARD A factor or exposure that may adversely affect health. A synonym for RISK.

HAZARD IDENTIFICATION See RISK ASSESSMENT.

HAZARD RATE (Syn: force of morbidity, instantaneous incidence rate) A theoretical measure of the risk of occurrence of an event, e.g., death, new disease, at a point in time, t, defined mathematically as the limit, as Δt approaches zero, of the probability that an individual well at time t will experience the event by $t + \Delta t$, divided by Δt.

HEALTH The World Health Organization (WHO) described *health* in 1948, in the preamble to its constitution, as "A state of complete physical, mental, and social well-being and not merely the absence of disease or infirmity." Noack[1] and many others have criticized the WHO description of health on the grounds that its terms are poorly defined and cannot be measured. In 1984, the WHO Health Promotion[2] initiative led to expansion of the original WHO description, which can be abbreviated to:

> The extent to which an individual or a group is able to realize aspirations and satisfy needs, and to change or cope with the environment. Health is a resource for everyday life, not the objective of living; it is a positive concept, emphasizing social and personal resources as well as physical capabilities.

Other definitions include the following:

> A state characterized by anatomic, physiologic and psychologic integrity; ability to perform personally valued family, work and community roles; ability to deal with physical, biologic, psychologic and social stress; a feeling of well-being; and freedom from the risk of disease and untimely death.[3]
>
> A state of equilibrium between humans and the physical, biologic and social environment, compatible with full functional activity.[4]

An ecological definition is:

> A state in which humans and other living creatures with which they interact can coexist indefinitely.

The word *health* is derived from the Old English *hal*, meaning whole, sound in wind and limb.

[1] Noack H. Concepts of Health and Health Promotion, in Abelin T, Brzeziński ZJ, Carstairs VDL, eds. *Measurement in Health Promotion and Protection.* Copenhagen: WHO, 1987:5–28.

[2] *Health Promotion: A Discussion Document.* Copenhagen: WHO, 1984.

[3] Stokes J III, Noren JJ, Shindell S. Definition of terms and concepts applicable to clinical preventive medicine. *J Commun Health* 1982; 8:33–41.

[4] Last JM. *Public Health and Human Ecology.* Norwalk, CT: Appleton and Lange, 1987:5.

HEALTH FOR ALL The objective of health care, enshrined in the Alma-Ata Declaration[1] (1978). It is interpreted as a goal to be achieved by the year 2000, or as a slogan or aspiration that might be realized by implementing primary health care for all the people of the world, or a country or region.

[1] Alma-Ata Declaration. Geneva and New York: WHO and UNICEF, 1978.

HEALTH-ADJUSTED LIFE EXPECTANCY Life expectancy expressed in quality-adjusted life years. See HEALTH EXPECTANCY.

HEALTH BEHAVIOR The combination of knowledge, practices, and attitudes that together contribute to motivate the actions we take regarding health. Health behavior
may promote and preserve good health, or if the behavior is harmful, e.g., tobacco
smoking, may be a determinant of disease. This combination of knowledge, practices, and attitudes has been described and discussed by several writers, notably
Becker.[1] See also ILLNESS BEHAVIOR.

[1] Becker MH, ed. *The Health Belief Model and Personal Health Behavior.* Thorofare NJ: Slack, 1974.

HEALTH CARE Services provided to individuals or communities by agents of the health
services or professions, promote, maintain, monitor, or restore health. Health care
is not limited to medical care, which implies therapeutic action by or under the
supervision of a physician. The term is sometimes extended to include self-care.

HEALTH EDUCATION The process by which individuals and groups of people learn to
behave in a manner conductive to the promotion, maintenance, or restoration of
health.

HEALTH EXPECTANCY The average amount of time (years, months, weeks, days) an
individual is expected to live in a given health state if current patterns of mortality
and health states continue to apply. A statistical abstraction based on existing age-
specific death rates and age-specific prevalences for health states, or age-specific
transition rates between health states.[1] *Health expectancy* is a general term, referring
to any one of a class of indicators. Specific health expectancies are based on health
states defined by ICIDH concepts of impairment, disability, and handicap. Examples include DISABILITY-FREE LIFE EXPECTANCY, HANDICAP-FREE LIFE EXPECTANCY.

[1] Robine JM, Mathers CD, Bucquet D. Distinguishing Health Expectancies and Health-Adjusted
Life Expectancies. *Am J Public Health* 1993; 83:797–798.

HEALTH INDEX A numerical indication of the health of a given population derived
from a specified composite formula. The components of the formula may be IN-
FANT MORTALITY RATES, INCIDENCE RATE for particular disease, or other HEALTH IN-
DICATOR.

HEALTH INDICATOR A variable, susceptible to direct measurement, that reflects the state
of health of persons in a community. Examples include infant mortality rates, incidence rates based on notified cases of disease, disability days, etc. These measures
may be used as components in the calculation of a HEALTH INDEX.

HEALTH PROMOTION The process of enabling people to increase control over and improve their health. It involves the population as a whole in the context of their
everyday lives, rather than focusing on people at risk for specific diseases, and is
directed toward action on the determinants or causes of health.[1]

[1] World Health Organization: *Ottawa Charter for Health Promotion.* Geneva: WHO, 1986.

HEALTH RISK APPRAISAL (HRA) (Syn: health hazard appraisal [HHA]) A generic term
applied to methods for describing an individual's chances of becoming ill or dying
from selected causes. The many versions available share several common features:
Starting from the average risk of death for the individual's age and sex, a consideration of various lifestyle and physical factors indicates whether the individual is at
greater or less than average risk of death from the commonest causes of death for
his age and sex. All methods also indicate what reduction in risk could be achieved
by altering any of the causal factors (such as cigarette smoking) that the individual
could modify.

　　The premise underlying such methods is that information on the extent to which
an individual's characteristics, habits, and health practices are influencing his future
risk of dying will assist health care workers in counseling their patients.

HEALTH SERVICES Services that are performed by health care professionals, or by others under their direction, for the purpose of promoting, maintaining, or restoring

health. In addition to personal health care, health services include measures for health protection, health promotion and disease prevention.

HEALTH SERVICES RESEARCH The integration of epidemiologic, sociological, economic, and other analytic sciences in the study of health services. Health services research is usually concerned with relationships between NEEDS, DEMAND, supply, use, and OUTCOMES of health services. The aim of health services research is evaluation; several components of evaluative health services research are distinguished, viz:

Evaluation of *structure*, concerned with resources, facilities, and manpower.

Evaluation of *process*, concerned with matters such as where, by whom, and how health care is provided.

Evaluation of *output*, concerned with the amount and nature of health services provided.

Evaluation of *outcome*, concerned with the results, i.e., whether persons using health services experience measurable benefits such as improved survival or reduced disability.

HEALTH STATISTICS Aggregated data describing and enumerating attributes, events, behaviors, services, resources, outcomes, or costs related to health, disease, and health services. The data may be derived from survey instruments, medical records, and administrative documents. VITAL STATISTICS are a subset of health statistics.

HEALTH STATUS The degree to which a person is able to function physically, emotionally, socially, with or without aid from the health care system. Compare QUALITY OF LIFE.

HEALTH STATUS INDEX A set of measurements designed to detect short-term fluctuations in the health of members of a population; these measurements include physical function, emotional well-being, activities of daily living, feelings, etc. Most indexes require the use of carefully composed questions designed with reference to matters of fact rather than shades of opinion. The results are usually expressed by a numerical score that gives a profile of the well-being of the individual.

HEALTH SURVEY A survey designed to provide information on the health status of a population. It may be descriptive, exploratory, or explanatory. See also MORBIDITY SURVEY, CROSS-SECTIONAL STUDY.

HEALTH SYSTEMS RESEARCH The coordinated study of determinants of health (nutrition, housing, employment, education, etc.) as well as factors directly associated with health, such as use and function of health services. A term popularized by the WHO.

HEALTHY WORKER EFFECT A phenomenon observed initially in studies of occupational diseases: Workers usually exhibit lower overall death rates than the general population, because the severely ill and chronically disabled are ordinarily excluded from employment. Death rates in the general population may be inappropriate for comparison if this effect is not taken into account.

HEALTHY YEAR EQUIVALENTS (HYES) A measure of health-related quality of life that incorporates two sets of preferences; one set reflects individuals' preferences for life years or duration of life; the other set reflects preferences for states of health.

HEBDOMADAL MORTALITY RATE The mortality rate in the first week of life; the denominator is the number of live births in a year.

HENLE–KOCH POSTULATES First formulated by F. G. Jacob Henle and adapted by Robert Koch in 1877, with elaborations in 1882. Koch stated that these postulates should be met before a causative relationship can be accepted between a particular bacterial parasite or disease agent and the disease in question.

1. The agent must be shown to be present in every case of the disease by isolation in pure culture.

2. The agent must not be found in cases of other disease.

3. Once isolated, the agent must be capable of reproducing the disease in experimental animals.

4. The agent must be recovered from the experimental disease produced.

See also CAUSALITY: EVANS'S POSTULATES, HILL'S CRITERIA.

HERD IMMUNITY The immunity of a group or community. The resistance of a group to invasion and spread of an infectious agent, based on the resistance to infection of a high proportion of individual members of the group. The resistance is a product of the number susceptible and the probability that those who are susceptible will come into contact with an infected person. Resistance of a population to invasion and spread of an infectious agent, based on the agent-specific immunity of a high proportion of the population. The proportion of the population required to be immune varies according to the agent, its transmission characteristics, the distribution of immunes and susceptibles, and other (e.g., environmental) factors.

HERD IMMUNITY THRESHOLD The proportion of immunes in a population, above which the incidence of the infection decreases.[1] This can be mathematically expressed as

$$H = 1 - 1/R_0 = (R_0 - 1)/R_0 = (rT - 1)/rT$$

where H is the herd immunity threshold, R_0 is the BASIC REPRODUCTIVE RATE, r is *the* TRANSMISSION PARAMETER, and T is the total population.

[1] Fine PEM. Herd immunity: History, theory, practice. *Epidemiol Rev* 1993; 15:265–302.

HERITABILITY The degree to which a trait is genetically determined, calculated by regression-correlation analyses among close relatives.

HETEROSCEDASTICITY Nonconstancy of the variance of a measure over the levels of the factors under study.

HEURISTIC METHOD A method of reasoning that relies on a combination of empirical observations and unproven theories to produce a solution that may be correct and defensible but cannot be proved. The word, not always perfectly understood by users or audience, sounds more impressive than the method. In common parlance, rule of thumb.

HIBERNATION Survival (of arthropod vectors) during cold periods.

HIERARCHY OF EVIDENCE The quality of epidemiologic evidence was appraised by the Canadian Task Force on the Periodic Health Examination[1] and the US Preventive Services Task Force[2] as an essential prerequisite to their recommendations about SCREENING and preventive interventions. The classes of evidence are:

I: Evidence from at least one properly designed randomized controlled trial.

II-1: Evidence from well-designed controlled trials without randomization.

II-2: Evidence from well-designed cohort or case control analytic studies, preferably from more than one center or research group.

II-3: Evidence obtained from multiple time series, with or without the intervention; dramatic results in uncontrolled experiments (e.g., first use of penicillin in the 1940s) also are in this category.

III: Opinions of respected authorities, based on clinical experience, descriptive studies, or reports of expert committees.

It is not always possible to achieve complete scientific rigor; for example, randomized controlled trials or cohort studies may be unethical or not feasible.

[1] Report of the Task Force on the Periodic Health Examination. *Can Med Assoc J* 1979; 121:1193–1254.

[2] *Guide to Clinical Preventive Services; Report of the U.S. Preventive Services Task Force.* Baltimore: Williams & Wilkins, 1989.

HILL'S CRITERIA OF CAUSATION The first complete statement of the epidemiologic criteria of a causal association is attributed to the British medical statistician Austin Bradford Hill[1] (1897–1991), although others[2] enunciated several of them. The criteria of a causal association of a factor and a disease are:

1. *Consistency:* The association is consistent when results are replicated in studies in different settings using different methods.
2. *Strength:* This is defined by the size of the risk as measured by appropriate statistical tests.
3. *Specificity:* This is established when a single putative cause produces a specific effect.
4. *Dose-response relationship:* An increasing level of exposure (in amount and/or time) increases the risk.
5. *Temporal relationship:* Exposure always precedes the outcome. This is the only absolutely essential criterion.
6. *Biological plausibility:* The association agrees with currently accepted understanding of pathobiological processes. This criterion should be applied with caution. As Sherlock Holmes remarked to Dr. Watson, "When you have eliminated the impossible, whatever remains, however improbable, must be the truth."
7. *Coherence:* The association should be compatible with existing theory and knowledge.
8. *Experiment:* The condition can be altered (e.g., prevented or ameliorated) by an appropriate experimental regimen.

[1] Hill AB. The environment and disease: Association or causation. *Proc R Soc Med* 1965; 58:295–300.
[2] Susser MW. What is a cause and how do we know one? A grammar for pragmatic epidemiology. *Am J Epidemiol* 1991; 133:635–648.

HISTOGRAM A graphic representation of the frequency distribution of a variable. Rectangles are drawn in such a way that their bases lie on a linear scale representing different intervals, and their heights are proportional to the frequencies of the values within each of the intervals. See also BAR DIAGRAM.

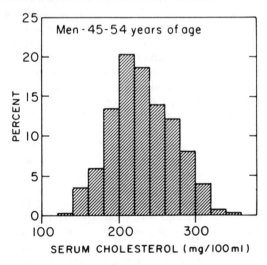

Histogram. Distribution of serum cholesterol levels in men aged 45–54.

HISTORICAL COHORT STUDY (Syn: historical prospective study, nonconcurrent prospective study, prospective study in retrospect) A COHORT STUDY conducted by reconstructing data about persons at a time or times in the past. This method uses existing records about the health or other relevant aspects of a population as it was at some time in the past and determines the current (or subsequent) status of members of this population with respect to the condition of interest. Different levels of past exposure to risk factor(s) of interest must be identifiable for subsets of the population. RECORD LINKAGE systems are often used in historical cohort studies. Growing public concern about protection of PRIVACY threatens such studies, which in the past have often made very valuable contributions to scientific understanding of disease causation. A DIRECTIVE of the European Community, if implemented, would make record linkage studies illegal.

HISTORICAL CONTROL Control subject(s) for whom data were collected at a time preceding that at which the data are gathered on the group being studied. Because of differences in exposure etc., use of historical controls can lead to bias in analysis.

HOGBEN NUMBER A unique personal identifying number constructed by using a sequence of digits for birth date, sex, birthplace, and other identifiers. Suggested by the English mathematician Lancelot Hogben. Used in primary care epidemiology in some countries and usable in RECORD LINKAGE. See also IDENTIFICATION NUMBER; SOUNDEX CODE.

HOLOENDEMIC DISEASE A disease for which a high prevalent level of infection begins early in life and affects most of the child population, leading to a state of equilibrium such that the adult population shows evidence of the disease much less commonly than do the children. Malaria in many communities is a holoendemic disease.

HOLOMIANTIC INFECTION See COMMON SOURCE EPIDEMIC.

HOMOSCEDASTICITY Constancy of the variance of a measure over the levels of the factors under study.

HOSPITAL-ACQUIRED INFECTION See NOSOCOMIAL INFECTION.

HOSPITAL DISCHARGE ABSTRACT SYSTEM Abstraction of MINIMUM DATA SET from hospital charts for the purpose of producing summary statistics about hospitalized patients. Examples include the Hospital Inpatient Enquiry (HIPE) and Professional Activity Study (PAS). The statistical tabulations commonly include length of stay by final diagnosis, surgical operations, specified hospital service (i.e., medical, surgical, gynecological, etc.) and also give outcomes such as "death" and "discharged alive from hospital." This system cannot generally be used for epidemiologic purposes as it is not possible to infer representativeness or to generalize; this is because the data usually lack a defined denominator and the same person may be counted more than once in the event of two or more HOSPITAL SEPARATIONS in the period of study. However, such data can be a fruitful source of cases for case control studies of rare conditions.

The systematic use of summary statistics on the process and outcome of hospital care began in the 19th century, pioneered in England by Florence Nightingale (1820–1910) and in Vienna by Ignaz Semmelweis (1818–1865). Nightingale was the founder of modern nursing care and an accomplished statistician—a member of the Royal Statistical Society. She was also a confrere of William Farr, Edwin Chadwick, and other great 19th century reformers. Her *Notes on Hospitals* (1859) discussed and illustrated the importance of statistical analysis of hospital activity. Semmelweis studied the outcome of obstetric care, demonstrating that puerperal sepsis was associated with attendance on women in labor by doctors who had come from the necropsy room to the labor room without washing their hands.

HOSPITAL INPATIENT ENQUIRY (HIPE) Statistical tables of a 10% sample of hospital patients in England and Wales, showing class of hospital, diagnosis, length of stay, outcomes, etc.

HOSPITAL SEPARATION A term used in commentaries on hospital statistics to describe the departure of a patient from hospital without distinguishing whether the patient departed alive or dead (the distinction is unimportant so far as the statistics of hospital activity such as bed occupancy are concerned).

HOST

1. A person or other living animal, including birds and arthropods, that affords subsistence or lodgment to an infectious agent under natural conditions. Some protozoa and helminths pass successive stages in alternate hosts of different species. Hosts in which the parasite attains maturity or passes its sexual stage are primary or definitive hosts; those in which the parasite is in a larval or asexual state are secondary or intermediate hosts. A transport host is a carrier in which the organism remains alive but does not undergo development.[1]

2. In an epidemiologic context, the host may be the population or group; biological, social, and behavioral characteristics of this group that are relevant to health are called "host factors."

[1] Benenson AS, ed. *Control of Communicable Diseases in Man*, 15th ed. Washington, DC: American Public Health Association, 1990.

HOST, DEFINITIVE In parasitology, the host in which sexual maturation occurs. In malaria, the mosquito (invertebrate host).

HOST, INTERMEDIATE In parasitology, the host in which asexual forms of the parasite develop. In malaria, this is a human or other vertebrate mammal or bird (vertebrate host).

HOUSEHOLD One or more persons who occupy a dwelling, i.e., a place that provides shelter, cooking, washing, and sleeping facilities; may or may not be a family. The term is also used to describe the dwelling unit in which the persons live.

HOUSEHOLD SAMPLE SURVEY A survey of persons in a sample of households. This, in many variations, is a favored method of gathering data for health-related and for many other purposes. The households may be sampled in any of several ways, e.g., by cluster, use of random numbers in relation to numbered dwelling units. The survey may be conducted by interview, telephone survey, or self-completed responses to present questions. The method is used in developing nations as well as in the industrial world.

HUMAN BLOOD INDEX Proportion of insect vectors found to contain human blood.

HUMAN DEVELOPMENT INDEX (HDI) A composite index combining indicators representing three dimensions—longevity (life expectancy at birth); knowledge (adult literacy rate and mean years of schooling); and income (real GDP per capita in purchasing-power-parity dollars). (Source: World Bank.)

HUMAN ECOLOGY See ECOLOGY.

HUMAN IMMUNODEFICIENCY VIRUS (HIV) The pathogenic organism responsible for the acquired immunodeficiency syndrome (AIDS); formerly or also known as the lymphadenopathy virus (LAV), the name given by the original French discoverers Montagnier et al.[1] in 1983, or the human T-cell lymphotropic virus, type III (HTLV-III), the name given by Gallo et al.[2] to the virus they reported in 1984. Retrovirus responsible for HIV disease, transmissible in blood, serum, semen, body tissues, other body fluids. The two main types, HIV-1 and HIV-2, attack T-helper lymphocytes, compromising immune responses to organisms that are destroyed by a healthy immune system. The virus is immunologically unstable, but it produces antibodies that can be detected by Western blot and ELISA tests of blood, serum, semen, saliva, etc.

[1] Barre-Sinoussi F, Cherman JC, Rey F, et al. Isolation of a T-lymphotropic retrovirus from a patient at risk for acquired immune deficiency syndrome (AIDS). *Science* 1983; 220:868–871.
[2] Gallo RC, Salahuddin SZ, Popovic M, et al. Frequent detection and isolation of cytopathic retroviruses (HTLV-III) from patients with AIDS and at risk for AIDS. *Science* 1984; 224:500–503.

HYPERENDEMIC DISEASE A disease that is constantly present at a high incidence and/or prevalence rate and affects all age groups equally.

HYPERGEOMETRIC DISTRIBUTION The exact probability distribution of the frequencies in a two-by-two contingency table, conditional on the marginal frequencies being fixed at their observed levels.

HYPOTHESIS

1. A supposition, arrived at from observation or reflection, that leads to refutable predictions.
2. Any conjecture cast in a form that will allow it to be tested and refuted.

See also NULL HYPOTHESIS.

I

IATROGENIC DISEASE Illness resulting from a physician's professional activity or from the professional activity of other health professionals.

ICD See INTERNATIONAL CLASSIFICATION OF DISEASE.

ICEBERG PHENOMENON That portion of disease which remains unrecorded or undetected despite physicians' diagnostic endeavors and community disease surveillance procedures is referred to as the "submerged portion of the iceberg." Detected or diagnosed disease is the "tip of the iceberg." The submerged portion comprises disease not medically attended, medically attended but not accurately diagnosed, and diagnosed but not reported.[1] Other terms have been proposed to describe this concept in parts of the world where icebergs are unknown, e.g., "ears of the hippopotamus," "crocodile's nose."

[1] Last JM. The iceberg. *Lancet* 1963; 2:28–31.

ICHPPC See INTERNATIONAL CLASSIFICATION OF HEALTH PROBLEMS IN PRIMARY CARE.

IDENTIFICATION NUMBER, IDENTIFYING NUMBER Unique number given to every individual at birth or at some other milestone. Sweden has a system based on a sequence of digits for birth date, sex, birthplace, and additional digits for each individual. Other systems, e.g., National Insurance number in the United Kingdom, Social Security number in the United States, and Social Insurance number in Canada, are sometimes used but are neither universal nor unique, being sometimes applied to whole families or at least to more than one individual. See also HOGBEN NUMBER; SOUNDEX CODE.

IDIOSYNCRASY Webster's Dictionary defines this as a distinctive characteristic or peculiarity of an individual. In PHARMACOEPIDEMIOLOGY, it means an abnormal reaction, sometimes genetically determined, following the administration of a medication.

ILLNESS The subjective state, or experience, of a person with DISEASE.

ILLNESS BEHAVIOR Conduct of persons in response to abnormal body signals. Such behavior influences the manner in which a person monitors his body, defines and interprets his symptoms, takes remedial actions, and uses the health care system. See also HEALTH BEHAVIOR.

IMMISSION Environmental concentration of a pollutant resulting from a combination of emissions and dispersals (often synonymous with EXPOSURE). (Source: IUPAC Glossary.)

IMMUNITY, ACQUIRED Resistance acquired by a host as a result of previous exposure to a natural PATHOGEN or foreign substance for the host, e.g., immunity to measles resulting from a prior infection with measles virus.

IMMUNITY, ACTIVE Resistance developed in response to stimulus by an antigen (infecting agent or vaccine) and usually characterized by the presence of antibody produced by the host.

IMMUNITY, NATURAL Species-determined inherent resistance to a disease agent, e.g., resistance of man to virus of canine distemper.

IMMUNITY, PASSIVE Immunity conferred by an antibody produced in another host and acquired naturally by an infant from its mother or artificially by administration of an antibody-containing preparation (antiserum or immune globulin).

IMMUNITY, SPECIFIC A state of altered responsiveness to a specific substance acquired through immunization or natural infection. For certain diseases (e.g., measles, chickenpox) this protection generally lasts for the life of the individual.

IMMUNIZATION (Syn: vaccination) Protection of susceptible individuals from communicable disease by administration of a living modified agent (as in yellow fever), a suspension of killed organisms (as in whooping cough), or an inactivated toxin (as in tetanus). Temporary passive immunization can be produced by administration of antibody in the form of immune globulin in some conditions.

IMMUNOGENICITY The ability of an infectious agent to induce specific immunity.

IMPACT FACTOR In SCIENTOMETRICS, a measure of the timeliness and frequency with which articles in a specific scientific periodical are cited by authors of articles in journals that are indexed in the Science Citation Index (SCI) and the Social Sciences Citation Index (SSCI).[1]

[1]Garfield E. Uses and misuses of citation frequency. *Current Contents* 1985; 43:3–9.

IMPACT FRACTION A generalization of POPULATION ATTRIBUTABLE RISK PERCENT that accommodates both hazardous and protective exposures, multiple levels of exposure, incomplete elimination of exposure, diffusion, or response to exposure. It is given by

$$\text{IF} = \frac{\Sigma(p'-p'')\text{RR}}{\Sigma p' \, \text{RR}} \quad \text{or} \quad \text{IF} = \frac{\Sigma(p''-p')}{\Sigma p' \, \text{RR}}$$

where IF = impact fraction, p' and p'' represent prevalences before and after an intervention program, and RR = Risk Ratio.

IMPAIRMENT A physical or mental defect at the level of a body system or organ. See also INTERNATIONAL CLASSIFICATION OF IMPAIRMENTS, DISABILITIES, AND HANDICAPS for the official WHO definition.

INAPPARENT INFECTION (Syn: subclinical infection) The presence of infection in a host without occurrence of recognizable clinical signs or symptoms. Of epidemiologic significance because hosts so infected, though apparently well, may serve as silent or inapparent disseminators of the infectious agent. See also DISEASE, PRECLINICAL; DISEASE, SUBCLINICAL; VECTOR-BORNE INFECTION.

INCEPTION COHORT A group of individuals identified for subsequent study at an early, uniform point in the course of the specified health condition, or before the condition develops. See also BASELINE DATA.

INCEPTION RATE The rate at which new spells of illness occur in a population; a term applied principally to short-term spells of illness such as acute respiratory infections, and preferred by some epidemiologists because an annual incidence rate for such conditions may exceed the numbers in the population at risk.

INCIDENCE (Syn: incident number) The number of instances of illness commencing, or of persons falling ill, during a given period in a specified population.[1] More generally, the number of new events, e.g., new cases of a disease in a defined population, within a specified period of time. The term incidence is sometimes used to denote INCIDENCE RATE.

[1]Prevalence and Incidence, *WHO Bull* 1966; 35:783–784.

INCIDENCE DENSITY The person-time incidence rate; sometimes used to describe the hazard rate. See FORCE OF MORBIDITY.

INCIDENCE-DENSITY RATIO (IDR) The ratio of two incidence densities. See also RATE RATIO.

INCIDENCE RATE The rate at which new events occur in a population. The numerator is the number of new events that occur in a defined period; the denominator is the population at risk of experiencing the event during this period, sometimes expressed as person-time. The incidence rate most often used in public health practice is calculated by the formula

$$\frac{\text{Number of new events in specified period}}{\substack{\text{Number of persons exposed to risk} \\ \text{during this period}}} \times 10^n$$

In a DYNAMIC POPULATION, the denominator is the average size of the population, often the estimated population at the mid-period. If the period is a year, this is the annual incidence rate. This rate is an estimate of the person-time incidence rate, i.e., the rate per 10^n person-years. If the rate is low, as with many chronic diseases, it is also a good estimate of the cumulative incidence rate. In follow-up studies with no CENSORING, the incidence rate is calculated by dividing the number of new cases in a specified period by the initial size of the cohort of persons being followed; this is equivalent to the cumulative incidence rate during the period. If the number of new cases during a specified period is divided by the sum of the person-time units at risk for all persons during the period, the result is the person-time incidence rate.

INCIDENCE STUDY See COHORT STUDY.

INCIDENT NUMBER See INCIDENCE.

INCUBATION PERIOD
1. The time interval between invasion by an infectious agent and appearance of the first sign or symptom of the disease in question. See also LATENT PERIOD.
2. In a VECTOR, the period between entry of the infectious agent into the vector and the time at which the vector becomes infective; i.e., transmission of the infectious agent from the vector to a fresh final host is possible (extrinsic incubation period).

INDEPENDENCE Two events are said to be independent if the occurrence of one is in no way predictable from the occurrence of the other. Two variables are said to be independent if the distribution of values of one is the same for all values of the other. *Independence* is the antonym of ASSOCIATION.

INDEPENDENT VARIABLE
1. The characteristic being observed or measured that is hypothesized to influence an event or manifestation (the dependent variable) within the defined area of relationships under study; that is, the independent variable is not influenced by the event or manifestation but may cause or contribute to variation of the event or manifestation.
2. In statistics, an independent variable is one of (perhaps) several variables that appear as arguments in a regression equation.

INDEX In epidemiology and related sciences, this word usually means a rating scale, e.g., a set of numbers derived from a series of observations of specified variables. Examples include the many varieties of health status index, scoring systems for severity or stage of cancer, heart murmurs, mental retardation, etc.

INDEX CASE The first case in a family or other defined group to come to the attention of the investigator. See also PROPOSITUS.

INDEX GROUP (Syn: index series)

1. In an experiment, the group receiving the experimental regimen.
2. In a case control study, the cases.
3. In a cohort study, the exposed group.

INDICATOR VARIABLE In statistics, a variable taking only one of two possible values, one (usually 1) indicating the presence of a condition, and the other (usually zero) indicating absence of the condition. Used mainly in REGRESSION ANALYSIS.

INDIRECT ADJUSTMENT See STANDARDIZATION.

INDIRECT OBSTETRIC DEATH See MATERNAL MORTALITY.

INDIRECT COSTS The value of resources lost. Indirect costs of morbidity include reduced levels of work output, time spent to obtain medical care, loss of productivity.[1]

[1] Rice D. Estimating the costs of illness. *Am J Public Health* 1967; 57:424–439.

INDIVIDUAL VARIATION Two types are distinguished:

1. *Intraindividual variation:* The variation of biological variables within the same individual, depending upon circumstances such as the phase of certain body rhythms and the presence or absence of emotional stress. These variables do not have a precise value, but rather a range. Examples include diurnal variation in body temperature, fluctuation of blood pressure, blood sugar, etc.
2. *Interindividual variation:* As used by Darwin, the term means variation *between* individuals. This is the preferred usage; the first usage is better described as personal variation.

INDUCTION Any method of logical analysis that proceeds from the particular to the general. No infallible method of logical reasoning exists, but general theories require induction. Conceptually bright ideas and breakthroughs and ordinary statistical inference belong to the realm of induction. Contrast DEDUCTION. See Medawar PB. *Induction and Intuition in Scientific Thought.* Philadelphia: American Philosophical Society, 1969.

INDUCTION PERIOD The period required for a specific cause to produce disease. More precisely, the interval from the causal action of a factor to the initiation of the disease. For example, a span of many years may pass between (presumably) radiation-induced mutations and the appearance of leukemia; this span would be the induction period for radiogenic leukemia. See also CARCINOGENESIS; INCUBATION PERIOD; LATENT PERIOD.

INDUSTRIAL HYGIENE The science and art devoted to recognition, evaluation, and control of those environmental factors or stresses arising from or in the workplace, which may cause sickness, impaired health, and well-being, or significant discomfort and inefficiency among workers or among persons in the community. Alternatively, the profession that anticipates and controls unhealthy conditions of work to prevent illness among employees. See also OCCUPATIONAL HEALTH.

INEQUALITIES IN HEALTH The virtually universal phenomenon of variation in health indicators (infant and maternal mortality rates, mortality and incidence rates of many diseases, etc.) associated with socioeconomic status. It has been observed since the vital statistics of England and Wales were examined by William Farr (1807–1883) and reported annually from 1840. If anything, the gap between best and worst health experience has widened in recent decades in the rich industrial nations like the USA and the UK. See, for example, Black D, Morris JN, Smith C, Townsend P. *Inequalities in Health.* Harmondsworth: Penguin, 1982; and Amler RW, Dull

HB, eds. *Closing the Gap: the Burden of Unnecessary Illness*. New York: Oxford University Press, 1987.

INFANT MORTALITY RATE (IMR) A measure of the yearly rate of deaths in children less than one year old. The denominator is the number of live births in the same year. Defined as

$$\text{Infant mortality rate} = \frac{\begin{array}{c}\text{Number of deaths in a year of}\\ \text{children less than 1 year of age}\end{array}}{\text{Number of live births in the same year}} \times 1000$$

This is often cited as a useful indicator of the level of health in a community.

INFECTIBILITY The host characteristic or state in which the host is capable of being infected. See also INFECTIOUSNESS; INFECTIVITY.

INFECTION (Syn: colonization) The entry and development or multiplication of an infectious agent in the body of man or animals. Infection is not synonymous with infectious disease; the result may be inapparent or manifest. The presence of living infectious agents on exterior surfaces of the body is called "infestation" (e.g., pediculosis, scabies). The presence of living infectious agents upon articles of apparel or soiled articles is not infection, but represents CONTAMINATION of such articles. See also INAPPARENT INFECTION; TRANSMISSION OF INFECTION.

INFECTION, GRADIENT OF The range of manifestations of illness in the host reflecting the response to an infectious agent, which extends from death at one extreme to inapparent infection at the other. The frequency of these manifestations varies with the specific infectious disease. For example, human infection with the virus of rabies is almost invariably fatal, whereas a high proportion of persons infected in childhood with the virus of hepatitis A, experience a subclinical or mild clinical infection.

INFECTION, LATENT PERIOD OF The time between initiation of infection and first shedding or excretion of the agent.

INFECTION, SUBCLINICAL See INAPPARENT INFECTION.

INFECTION RATE The incidence rate of manifest plus inapparent infections (the latter determined by seroepidemiology).

INFECTION TRANSMISSION PARAMETER (r) The proportion of total possible contacts between infectious cases and susceptibles which lead to new infections.

INFECTIOUS DISEASE See COMMUNICABLE DISEASE.

INFECTIOUSNESS A characteristic of a disease that concerns the relative ease with which it is transmitted to other hosts. A droplet spread disease, for instance, is more infectious than one spread by direct contact. The characteristics of the portals of exit and entry are thus also determinants of infectiousness, as are the agent characteristics of ability to survive away from the host, and of infectivity.

INFECTIVITY
1. The characteristic of the disease agent that embodies capability to enter, survive, and multiply in the host. A measure of infectivity is the secondary attack rate.
2. The proportion of exposures, in defined circumstances, that results in infection.

INFERENCE The process of passing from observations and axioms to generalizations. In statistics, the development of generalization from sample data, usually with calculated degrees of uncertainty.

INFESTATION The development on (rather than in) the body of a pathogenic agent, e.g., body lice. Some authors use the term also to describe invasion of the gut by parasitic worms.

INFORMATICS The study of information and the ways to handle it, especially by means of information technology, i.e., computers and other electronic devices for rapid transfer, processing, and analysis of large amounts of data. See *Informatics and Telematics in Health*. Geneva: WHO, 1988.

INFORMATION BIAS (Syn: observational bias) A flaw in measuring exposure or outcome data that results in different quality (accuracy) of information between comparison groups.

INFORMATION SUPERHIGHWAY (jargon) The electronic transmission of data, information, ideas, and pictures among computers via modems, fiberoptic cables, satellite communication, etc. The communication network of computers is the *Internet*[1] and a popular mode of use is electronic mail, or *e-mail*. The rapid growth of this form of communication is remarkable; as of mid-1994, it linked an estimated 14 million users worldwide. It provides online access to information in current medical journals[2] and capability to search the catalogues of some of the world's largest libraries (e.g., the National Library of Medicine).[3] The tables of contents and abstracts of articles published in journals listed in the *Index Medicus* and other retrieval systems are accessible on computer terminals using programs such as Medline, Grateful-Med, and Epi-Info. In disease surveillance and control, the Internet can be used for instantaneous worldwide reporting of epidemic outbreaks.[4]

[1] Krol E. *The Whole Internet*. Sebastopol, CA: O'Reilly and Associates, 1992.

[2] Glowniak JV, Bushway MK. Computer networks as a medical resource: Accessing and using the Internet. *JAMA* 1994; 271:1934–1939.

[3] Laporte RE, Akazawa S, Hellmonds P et al. Global public health and the information superhighway. *Br Med J* 1994; 308:1651–1652.

[4] Laporte RE, Gooch WA, Gamboa C, Tajima N. International disease counting (IDC) form. *Lancet* 1993; 342:930–931.

INFORMATION SYSTEM A combination of vital and health statistical data from multiple sources, used to derive information about the health needs, health resources, costs, use of health services, and outcomes of use by the population of a specified jurisdiction. The term may also describe the automatic release from computers of stored information in response to programmed stimuli. For example, parents can be notified when their children are due to receive booster doses of an immunizing agent against infectious disease.

INFORMATION THEORY Mathematical theory dealing with the nature, effectiveness, and accuracy of information transfer.

INFORMED CONSENT Voluntary consent given by a subject—i.e., person or a responsible proxy (e.g., a parent)—for participation in a study, immunization program, treatment regimen, etc., after being informed of the purpose, methods, procedures, benefits and risks, and, when relevant, the degree of uncertainty about outcome. The essential criteria of informed consent are that the subject has both knowledge and comprehension, that consent is freely given without duress or undue influence, and that the right of withdrawal at any time is clearly communicated to the subject. Other aspects of informed consent in the context of epidemiologic and biomedical research, and criteria to be met in obtaining it, are specified in *International Guidelines for Ethical Review of Epidemiological Studies* (Geneva: CIOMS/WHO 1991) and *International Ethical Guidelines for Biomedical Research Involving Human Subjects* (Geneva: CIOMS/WHO 1993).

INGELFINGER RULE Rule developed by Franz Ingelfinger (1910–1980) former editor of the *New England Journal of Medicine,* as follows:

The Journal undertakes review with the understanding that neither the substance of the article nor the figures or tables have been published or will be submitted for publication during the period of review. This restriction does not apply to abstracts published in connection with scientific meetings or to news reports based on public presentations at such meetings.[1]

A revision of the rule imposes a news embargo[2] until the pertinent article is published. The Ingelfinger rule (or modifications of it) has been adopted by many high-quality peer-reviewed biomedical science journals. The aims of the rule are to eliminate duplicate publication and reduce uncritical acceptance of original work prior to peer review and publication.

[1] Relman AS. The Ingelfinger Rule. *N Engl J Med* 1981; 305:824–826.
[2] Angell M, Kassirer JP. The Ingelfinger Rule revisited. *N Engl J Med* 1991; 325:1371–1373.

INOCULATION See VACCINATION.

INPUT

1. The sum total of resources and energies purposefully engaged in order to intervene in the spontaneous operation of a system.
2. The basic resources required in terms of manpower, money, materials, and time.

INSTANTANEOUS INCIDENCE RATE See FORCE OF MORBIDITY.

INSTITUTIONAL REVIEW BOARD (IRB) The term used in the USA to describe the standing committee in a medical school, hospital, or other health care facility that is charged with ensuring the safety and well-being of human subjects involved in research. The IRB is responsible for ethical review of research proposals. Many synonyms are used in other countries, e.g., *Ethical Review Committee, Research Ethics Board.* All research, including epidemiologic research, that involves human subjects must be approved by an Institutional Review Board or equivalent body.

INSTRUMENTAL ERROR Error due to faults arising in any or in all aspects of a measuring instrument, i.e., calibration, accuracy, precision, etc. Also applied to error arising from impure reagents, wrong dilutions, etc.

INTENTION-TO-TREAT ANALYSIS A procedure[1] in the conduct and analysis of randomized controlled trials. All patients allocated to each arm of the treatment regimen are analyzed together as representing that treatment arm, whether or not they received or completed the prescribed regimen. Failure to follow this step defeats the main purpose of RANDOM ALLOCATION and can invalidate the results.

[1] Newell DJ. Editorial, *Int J Epidemiol* 1992; 21:837–841.

INTERACTION

1. The interdependent operation of two or more causes to produce or prevent an effect. *Biological interaction* means the interdependent operation of two or more causes to produce, prevent, or control disease. See also ANTAGONISM; SYNERGISM.
2. Differences in the effects of one or more factors according to the level of the remaining factor(s). See also EFFECT MODIFIER.
3. In statistics, the necessity for a product term in a linear model.

INTERMEDIATE VARIABLE (Syn: contingent variable, intervening [causal] variable, mediator variable) A variable that occurs in a causal pathway from an independent to a dependent variable. It causes variation in the dependent variable, and itself is caused to vary by the independent variable. Such a variable is statistically associated with both the independent and dependent variables.

INTERNAL VALIDITY See VALIDITY, STUDY.

INTERNATIONAL CLASSIFICATION OF DISEASE (ICD) The classification of specific conditions and groups of conditions determined by an internationally representative group of experts who advise the World Health Organization, which publishes the complete list in periodic revisions. Every disease entity is assigned a number. There are 21 major divisions *(chapters)* and a hierarchical arrangement of subdivisions *(rubrics)* within each in the tenth revision. Some chapters are "etiologic," e.g., Infective and Parasitic Conditions; others relate to body systems, e.g., Circulatory System; and some to classes of condition, e.g., neoplasms, injury (violence). The heterogeneity of categories reflects prevailing uncertainties about causes of disease (and classification in relation to causes). The tenth revision of the manual *(ICD-10)* was published by WHO in 1990, after ratification in 1989. See also INTERNATIONAL STATISTICAL CLASSIFICATION OF DISEASES AND RELATED HEALTH PROBLEMS (ICD-10).

INTERNATIONAL CLASSIFICATION OF HEALTH PROBLEMS IN PRIMARY CARE (ICHPPC) A classification of diseases, conditions, and other reasons for attendance for primary care. May be used for labeling conditions in problem-oriented records as used by primary care health workers. This classification is an adaptation of the ICD but makes more allowance for the diagnostic uncertainty that prevails in primary care. This classification is now in its second revision (ICHPPC-2). See also PROBLEM-ORIENTED MEDICAL RECORD.

INTERNATIONAL CLASSIFICATION OF IMPAIRMENTS, DISABILITIES, AND HANDICAPS (ICIDH) First published by WHO in 1980, this is an attempt to produce a systematic taxonomy of the consequences of injury and disease.

An *impairment* is defined in ICIDH as any loss or abnormality of psychological, physiological, or anatomical structure or function. It is concerned with abnormalities of body structure and appearance and with organ or system function resulting from any cause; in principle, impairments represent disturbances at the organ level.

A *disability* is defined in ICIDH as any restriction or lack (resulting from an impairment) of ability to perform an activity in a manner or within the range considered normal for a human being. The term disability reflects the consequences of impairment in terms of functional performance and activity by the individual; disabilities thus represent disturbances at the level of the person.

A *handicap* is defined in ICIDH as a disadvantage for a given individual, resulting from an impairment or a disability, that limits or prevents the fulfillment of a role that is normal (depending on age, sex, and social and cultural practice) for that individual. The term handicap thus reflects interaction with and adaptation to the individual's surroundings.

INTERNATIONAL CLASSIFICATION OF PRIMARY CARE (ICPC) The official classification of the World Organization of Family Doctors (WONCA).[1] It includes three elements of the doctor-patient encounter: the REASON FOR ENCOUNTER (RFE), the diagnosis, and the treatment or other action or intervention. It is a biaxial classification system based on chapters and components. It uses three-digit alphanumeric codes with mnemonic qualities to facilitate its day-to-day use. Seventeen chapters, each with an alpha code, form one axis; seven components with rubrics having a two-digit numeric code form the second axis. The components deal with symptoms and complaints, diagnoses and therapeutic interventions, administrative procedures and diseases. The ICPC has been converted to *ICD-9* and *ICD-10*.

[1] Lamberts H, Wood M, ed. *ICPC, International Classification of Primary Care.* Oxford, England, New York: Oxford Medical Publications, 1987.

INTERNATIONAL COMPARISONS Arranging the nations of the world in tables that show the rank order of vital statistics such as infant mortality rates, death or incidence rates for cancer, heart disease, etc. This is a popular pastime of polemicists and politicians, but international comparisons must be interpreted cautiously. The dangers of making comparisons include the shifting tides of diagnostic fashion and the varying criteria and definitions that prevail from one nation to another. Only after ensuring that like is truly being compared with like can the comparisons be trusted and, even then, with reservations about validity. See also CROSS-CULTURAL STUDY.

INTERNATIONAL FORM OF MEDICAL CERTIFICATE OF CAUSES OF DEATH In adopting the tenth revision of *ICD* in 1990, the World Health Assembly resolved that causes of death to be entered on the medical certificate of cause of death are all those diseases, morbid conditions, or injuries that either resulted in or contributed to death and the circumstances of the accident or violence that produced such injuries. Antecedent causes and other significant conditions are also to be recorded. See also DEATH CERTIFICATE.

INTERNATIONAL NOMENCLATURE OF DISEASES (IND) Since 1970, the Council for International Organizations of the Medical Sciences (CIOMS) and WHO have collaborated in preparing an International Nomenclature of Diseases (IND). This is a complement to the ICD. The purpose of the IND is to provide a single recommended name for every disease entity. The criteria for selection are that the name should be specific, unambiguous, as self-descriptive and as simple as possible, and based on cause whenever feasible. A list of synonyms is appended to each definition.

INTERNATIONAL STATISTICAL CLASSIFICATION OF DISEASES AND RELATED HEALTH PROBLEMS The tenth revision, known in short as *ICD-10*, was approved by the International Conference for the Tenth Revision in 1989 and by the 43rd World Health Assembly in 1990. It is the latest in a series of international classifications dating back to the BERTILLON CLASSIFICATION (i.e., the International List of Causes of Death, 1893); *ICD-10* came into effect at the beginning of 1993, exactly 100 years after the original. The tenth revision has 21 chapters and uses an alphanumeric coding system in order to provide a larger coding frame than previously, leaving room for future expansion. The chapters of *ICD-10* are as follows:

I (A00–B99): Certain infectious and parasitic diseases

II (C00–D97): Neoplasms

III (D50–D89): Diseases of the blood and blood-forming organs and certain disorders involving the immune mechanism

IV (E00–E90): Endocrine, nutritional, and metabolic diseases

V (F00–F99): Mental and behavioral disorders

VI (G00–G99): Diseases of the nervous system

VII (H00–H59): Diseases of the eye and adnexa

VIII (H60–H95): Diseases of the ear and mastoid process

IX (I00–I99): Diseases of the circulatory system

X (J00–J99): Diseases of the respiratory system

XI (K00–K93): Diseases of the digestive system

XII (L00–L99): Diseases of the skin and subcutaneous tissue

XIII (M00–M99): Diseases of the musculoskeletal system and connective tissue

XIV (N00–N99): Diseases of the genitourinary system

XV (O00–O99): Pregnancy, childbirth, and the puerperium

XVI (P00–P96): Certain conditions originating in the perinatal period

XVII (Q00–Q99): Congenital malformations, deformations, and chromosomal abnormalities

XVIII (R00–R99): Symptoms, signs, and abnormal clinical and laboratory findings not elsewhere classified

XIX (S00–T98): Injury, poisoning, and certain other consequences of external causes

XX (V01–Y99): External causes of morbidity and mortality

XXI (Z00–Z99): Factors influencing health status and contact with health services

INTERNET See INFORMATION SUPERHIGHWAY.

INTERPOLATE, INTERPOLATION To predict the value of variates within the range of observations; the resulting prediction.

INTERSECTORAL COLLABORATION A term used mainly in UN agencies to describe activities involving several components of the body politic—e.g., the health sector, the education sector, the housing sector—that working together can enhance health conditions more effectively than when working independently of one another.

INTERVAL The set containing all numbers between two given numbers.

INTERVAL INCIDENCE DENSITY See PERSON-TIME INCIDENCE RATE.

INTERVAL SCALE See MEASUREMENT SCALE.

INTERVENING CAUSE See INTERMEDIATE VARIABLE.

INTERVENING VARIABLE

1. Synonym for INTERMEDIATE VARIABLE.
2. A variable whose value is altered in order to block or alter the effect(s) of another factor.

See also CAUSALITY.

INTERVENTION INDEX An estimate of the impact of a therapeutic or preventive intervention.[1] It is the ratio of (1) the number of persons whose risk level must change to prevent one premature death to (2) the total number at risk.

[1] Rothenburg R, Ford ES, Vaitianen R: Ischemic heart disease: estimating the impact of interventions. *J Clin Epidemiol* 1992; 45:1:21–29.

INTERVENTION STUDY An investigation involving intentional change in some aspect of the status of the subjects, e.g., introduction of a preventive or therapeutic regimen, or designed to test a hypothesized relationship; usually an EXPERIMENT such as a RANDOMIZED CONTROLLED TRIAL.

INTERVIEW SCHEDULE The precisely designed set of questions used in an interview. See also SURVEY INSTRUMENT.

INTERVIEWER BIAS Systematic error due to interviewers' subconscious or conscious gathering of selective data.

INVOLUNTARY SMOKING (Syn: passive smoking) The inhalation by nonsmokers of tobacco smoke left in the air by smokers (ENVIRONMENTAL TOBACCO SMOKE); includes both smoke exhaled by smokers and smoke released directly from burning tobacco into ambient air; the latter is called SIDESTREAM SMOKE and contains higher proportions of toxic and other carcinogenic substances than exhaled smoke. The adjective *involuntary* is preferable to *passive* as the latter implies acquiescence—increasingly, nonsmokers are anything but acquiescent about this form of air pollution.

ISLAND POPULATION A group of individuals isolated from larger groups and possessing a relatively limited gene pool; alternatively, a group that is immunologically isolated and may therefore be unduly susceptible to infection with alien pathogens.

ISODEMOGRAPHIC MAP (Syn: density-equalizing map) A diagrammatic method of displaying administrative jurisdictions of a country in two-dimensional "maps" with areas directly proportional to the population density of the jurisdictions. Thus densely populated urban regions occupy large areas of the map and sparsely inhabited rural regions occupy small areas. Additional data—such as incidence or mortality rates within each jurisdiction—can be superimposed in colors or shading to represent rates.

ISOLATE (noun) Term used in genetics to describe a subpopulation (generally small) in which matings take place exclusively with other members of the same subpopulation.

ISOLATION

1. In microbiology, the separation of an organism from others, usually by making serial cultures.

2. Separation, for the period of communicability, of infected persons or animals from others in such places and under such conditions as to prevent or limit the direct or indirect transmission of the infectious agent from those infected to those who are susceptible or who may spread the agent to others. *CDC Guidelines for Isolation Precautions in Hospitals* (1990) expanded on blood and body fluid precautions described below. *Control of Communicable Disease in Man*[1] lists seven categories of isolation as follows:

   a. *Strict isolation:* This category is designed to prevent transmission of highly contagious or virulent infections that may be spread by both air and contact. The specifications, in addition to those above, include a private room and the use of masks, gowns, and gloves for all persons entering the room. Special ventilation requirements with the room at negative pressure to surrounding areas are desirable.

   b. *Contact isolation:* For less highly transmissible or serious infections, for diseases or conditions that are spread primarily by close or direct contact. In addition to the basic requirements, a private room is indicated but patients infected with the same pathogen may share a room. Masks are indicated for those who come close to the patient, gowns are indicated if soiling is likely, and gloves are indicated for touching infectious material.

   c. *Respiratory isolation:* To prevent transmission of infectious diseases over short distances through the air, a private room is indicated but patients infected with the same organism may share a room. In addition to the basic requirements, masks are indicated for those who come in close contact with the patient; gowns and gloves are not indicated.

   d. *Tuberculosis isolation (AFB isolation):* For patients with pulmonary tuberculosis who have a positive sputum smear or chest x-rays that strongly suggest active tuberculosis. Specifications include use of a private room with special ventilation and the door closed. In addition to the basic requirements, masks are used only if the patient is coughing and does not reliably and consistently cover the mouth. Gowns are used to prevent gross contamination of clothing. Gloves are not indicated.

   e. *Enteric precautions:* For infections transmitted by direct or indirect contact with feces. In addition to the basic requirements, specifications include use of a private room if patient hygiene is poor. Masks are not indicated; gowns should be used if soiling is likely and gloves are to be used for touching contaminated materials.

   f. *Drainage/secretion precautions:* To prevent infections transmitted by direct or indirect contact with purulent material or drainage from an infected body site. A private room and masking are not indicated; in addition to the basic requirements, gowns should be used if soiling is likely and gloves used for touching contaminated materials.

g. *Blood/body fluid precautions:* To prevent infections that are transmitted by direct or indirect contact with infected blood or body fluids. In addition to the basic requirements, a private room is indicated if patient hygiene is poor; masks are not indicated; gowns should be used if soiling of clothing with blood or body fluids is likely. Gloves should be used for touching blood or body fluids. Blood and body fluid precautions should be used consistently for all patients regardless of their blood-borne infection status ("universal blood and body fluid precautions"). These are intended to pre-vent parenteral, mucous membrane, and nonintact-skin exposure of health care workers to blood-borne pathogens. Protective barriers include gloves, gowns, masks, and protective eyewear. See also UNIVERSAL PRECAUTIONS.

See also QUARANTINE.

[1]Benenson AS, ed. *Control of Communicable Diseases in Man,* 15th ed. Washington DC: American Public Health Association, 1990.

ISOMETRIC CHART A chart or graph that portrays three dimensions on a plane surface.

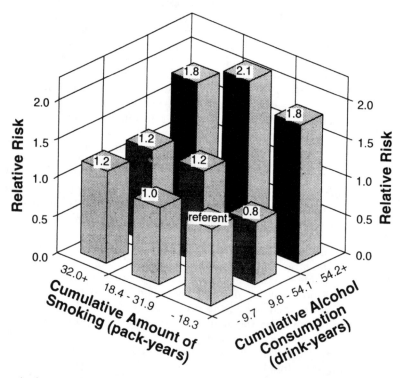

Isometric chart. Relative risks of hepatocellular carcinoma according to cumulative alco-hol consumption and amount of smoking. From Tanaka K, Hirohata T: *Japan J Epide-mial* 1992; 2:2 (Suppl): S-167. With permission.

J, K

JACKKNIFE A technique for estimating the variance and the bias of an estimator. If the sample size is n, the estimator is applied to each subsample of size $n-1$, obtained by dropping a measurement from analysis. The sum of squared differences between each of the resulting estimates and their mean, multiplied by $(n-1)/n$, is the jackknife estimate of variance; the difference between the mean and the original estimate, multiplied by $(n-1)$, is the jackknife estimate of bias.

JARMAN SCORE An index of communitywide social deprivation, used mainly by general practitioners in the UK.[1] Unlike the TOWNSEND SCORE, the Jarman score has no theoretical basis; it uses weighted values for percentages of elderly persons living alone; children aged under 5 years; single-parent families; social class V (unskilled workers); unemployed; overcrowded dwellings; changed address in the past year; ethnic minorities. The Jarman score correlates quite well with other indices as a measure of group socioeconomic status in administratively defined jurisdictions such as urban areas, but is not universally accepted as a valid index. See also OVERCROWDING, TOWNSEND SCORE.

[1] Jarman B. Identification of underprivileged areas. *Br Med J* 1983; 286:1075–1079.

JELLINEK FORMULA A formula to estimate the prevalence of alcohol-related disease, based on the assumption that a predictable proportion of persons addicted to alcohol die of cirrhosis of the liver (confirmed by necropsy). The formula fails to allow for biases, e.g., in autopsy series, for the frequency of other causes of cirrhosis and for variations in the dose response and end organ damage produced by alcohol abuse; it is therefore flawed.

JONES CRITERIA Set of clinical and laboratory findings for the diagnosis of rheumatic fever. The criteria include presence of group A hemolytic streptococcal infection; major manifestations (carditis, polyarthritis, etc.); minor manifestations (fever, arthralgia, etc.); ancillary tests (raised erythrocyte sedimentation rate, C-reactive protein, etc.).

KAP (KNOWLEDGE, ATTITUDES, PRACTICE) SURVEY A formal survey, using face-to-face interviews, in which women are asked standardized pretested questions dealing with their knowledge of, attitudes toward, and use of contraceptive methods. Detailed reproductive histories and attitudes toward desired family size are also elicited. Analysis of responses provides much useful information on family planning and gives estimates of possible future trends in population structure. The term has sometimes been used to describe other varieties of survey of knowledge, attitudes, and practice, e.g., health promotion in general or in particular, cigarette smoking.

KAPLAN-MEIER ESTIMATE (Syn: product limit method) A nonparametric method of compiling life or survival tables, developed by Kaplan and Meier in 1958. This combines calculated probabilities of survival and estimates to allow for CENSORED observations, which are assumed to occur randomly. The intervals are defined as ending each time an event (death, withdrawal) occurs and are therefore unequal.

KAPPA A measure of the degree of nonrandom agreement between observers or measurements of the same categorical variable

$$k = \frac{P_0 - P_e}{1 - P_e}$$

where P_0 is the proportion of times the measurements agree, and P_e is the proportion of times they can be expected to agree by chance alone. If the measurements agree more often than expected by chance, kappa is positive; if concordance is complete, kappa$= 1$; if there is no more nor less than chance concordance, kappa$= 0$; if the measurements disagree more than expected by chance, kappa is negative.

KENDALL'S TAU See CORRELATION COEFFICIENT.

KOCH'S POSTULATES See HENLE-KOCH POSTULATES. See also CAUSALITY; EVANS'S POSTULATES.

KRIGING A method first used in the earth sciences to smooth data from spatially scattered point measurements, e.g., drill sites. It is used in geographic epidemiology.[1] The method relies on analysis of the spatial variability of the data and allows representation of the variable under study as a continuous process throughout the country. The method is named for its developer, D. G. Krige.

[1] Carrat F, Valleron A-J. Epidemiologic mapping using the "Kriging" method: application to an influenza-like illness in France. *Am J Epidemiol* 1992; 135:1293–1300.

KURTOSIS The extent to which a unimodal distribution is peaked.

L

LARGE SAMPLE METHOD (Syn: asymptotic method) Any statistical method based on an approximation to a normal or other distribution that becomes more accurate as sample size increases. An example is a chi square test on a set of frequencies.

LATE MATERNAL DEATH See MATERNAL MORTALITY.

LATENT HETEROGENEITY Epidemiologic data that are too heterogeneous to be described by a simple mathematical model such as the binomial or Poisson distribution, suggestive of the effect of unidentified risk factors.

LATENT IMMUNIZATION The process of developing immunity by a single or repeated inapparent asymptomatic infection. Not necessarily related to latent infection. See also IMMUNITY, ACQUIRED.

LATENT INFECTION Persistence of an infectious agent within the host without symptoms (and often without demonstrable presence in blood, tissues, or bodily secretions of host).

LATENT PERIOD (Syn: latency) Delay between exposure to a disease-causing agent and the appearance of manifestations of the disease. After exposure to ionizing radiation, for instance, there is a latent period of 5 years, on average, before development of leukemia, and more than 20 years before development of certain other malignant conditions. The term *latent period* is often used synonymously with *induction period*, that is, the period between exposure to a disease-causing agent and the appearance of manifestations of the disease. It has also been defined as the period from disease initiation to disease detection. In infectious disease epidemiology, this corresponds to the period between exposure and the onset of infectiousness (this may be shorter or longer than the incubation period). See also INCUBATION PERIOD; INDUCTION PERIOD.

LATIN SQUARE One of the basic statistical designs for experiments that aim at removing from the experimental error the variation from two sources, which may be identified with the rows and columns of the square. In such a design the allocation of k experimental treatments in the cells of a k by k (latin) square is such that each treatment occurs exactly once in each row and column. A design for a 5×5 square is as follows:

A	B	C	D	E
B	A	E	C	D
C	D	A	E	B
D	E	B	A	C
E	C	D	B	A

After Kendall and Buckland.[1]

[1] Kendall MG, Buckland AA. *A Dictionary of Statistical Terms,* 4th ed. London: Longman, 1982.

LAW OF LARGE NUMBERS This law, enunciated by Jacob Bernoulli (1654–1705) states that the accuracy of a sample mean is increased (or the standard error of a statistic is reduced) as the numbers studied increase. In other words, the larger the sample, the more likely it is to be representative of the "universe" population.

LEAD TIME The time gained in treating or controlling a disease when detection is earlier than usual, e.g., in the presymptomatic stage, as when screening procedures are used for detection.

LEAD TIME BIAS (Syn: zero time shift) Overestimation of survival time, due to the backward shift in the starting point for measuring survival that arises when diseases such as cancer are detected early, as by screening procedures. More generally, a systematic error arising when follow-up of groups does not begin at comparable stages in the natural history of a condition. For example, interventions for women whose breast cancer is detected by screening cannot be validly compared with interventions for women whose disease is first detected by clinical examination at a later stage of the disease. See also ZERO-TIME SHIFT.

LEAST SQUARES A principle of estimation, due to Gauss, in which the estimates of a set of parameters in a statistical model are those quantities that minimize the sum of squared differences between the observed values of the dependent variable and the values predicted by the model.

LEDERMANN FORMULA Ledermann[1] showed empirically that the frequency distribution of alcohol consumption in the population of consumers may be log-normal; the curve is sharply skewed—approximately one-third of drinkers consume more than 60% of the total amount of alcohol. Among drinkers the proportion of persons with alcoholism remains constant at around 7–9%. The pattern of consumption of illicit drugs among users may also be log-normal. Questions have been raised, however, about the validity of some assumptions upon which the formula is based.

[1] Ledermann S. *Alcool, Alcoolisme et Alcoolisation.* Paris: Presses universitaires de France, 1956.

LENGTH BIAS A systematic error due to selection of disproportionate numbers of long-duration cases (cases who survive longest) in one group but not in another. This can occur when prevalent rather than incident cases are included in a case control study.

LEVIN'S ATTRIBUTABLE RISK See ATTRIBUTABLE FRACTION (POPULATION).

LIFE EVENTS Aspects of the pattern of living that may be associated with or produce changes in health. The relationship of "life stress" and "emotional stress" to onset of several kinds of serious chronic disease such as coronary heart disease and hypertension has been the subject of epidemiologic studies. The Rahe-Holmes Social Readjustment Rating Scale[1] was the first to be developed to assign ranks or ratings to significant life events such as death of a spouse or other close relative, loss of regular job, relocation, marriage, divorce, etc. Many other rating scales have since been developed.

[1] Holmes TH, Rahe RH: The social readjustment rating scale. *J Psychosom Res* 1967; 1:213–218.

LIFE EXPECTANCY See EXPECTATION OF LIFE.

LIFE EXPECTANCY FREE FROM DISABILITY (LEFD) An estimate of life expectancy adjusted for activity-limitation (data for which are derived from hospital discharge statistics, etc.). See DISABILITY-FREE LIFE EXPECTANCY, QALY.

LIFE EXPECTANCY WITH DISABILITY The average number of years an individual is expected to live with disability if current patterns of mortality and disability continue to apply. See DISABILITY-FREE LIFE EXPECTANCY.

LIFE-STYLE The set of habits and customs that is influenced, modified, encouraged, or constrained by the lifelong process of socialization. These habits and customs include use of substances such as alcohol, tobacco, tea, coffee; dietary habits, exercise, etc., which have important implications for health and are often the subject of epidemiologic investigations.

LIFE TABLE A summarizing technique used to describe the pattern of mortality and survival in populations. The survival data are time specific and cumulative probabilities of survival of a group of individuals subject, throughout life, to the age-specific death rates in question. The life table method can be applied to the study not only of death, but also of any defined endpoint such as the onset of disease or the occurrence of specific complication(s) of disease. The survivors to age x are denoted by the symbol l_x, the expectation of life at age x is denoted by the symbol $\mathring{e}_x$, and the proportion alive at age x who die between age x and $x+1$ years is denoted by the symbol nq_x. The life table method is used extensively in epidemiology and in many assessments of treatment regimens in clinical practice.

The first rudimentary life tables were published in 1693 by the astronomer Edmund Halley. These made use of records of the funerals in the city of Breslau. In 1815 in England, the first actuarially correct life table was published, based on both population and death data classified by age.

Two types of life tables may be distinguished according to the reference year of the table: the current or period life table and the generation or cohort life table.

The current life table is a summary of mortality experience over a brief period (one to three years), and the population data relate to the middle of that period (usually close to the date of a census). A current life table therefore represents the combined mortality experience by age of the population in a particular short period of time.

The cohort or generation life table describes the actual survival experience of a group, or cohort, of individuals born at about the same time. Theoretically, the mortality experience of the persons in the cohort would be observed from their moment of birth through each consecutive age in successive calendar years until all of them die.

The clinical life table describes the outcome experience of a group or cohort of individuals classified according to their exposure or treatment history.

Life tables are also classified according to the length of age interval in which the data are presented. A complete life table contains data for every single year of age from birth to the last applicable age. An abridged life table contains data by intervals of 5 or 10 years of age. See also EXPECTATION OF LIFE; SURVIVORSHIP STUDY.

LIFE TABLE, EXPECTATION OF LIFE FUNCTION, $\mathring{e}_x$ (Syn: average future lifetime) The expectation of life function is a statement of the average number of years of life remaining to persons who survive to age x.

LIFE TABLE, SURVIVORSHIP FUNCTION, l_x The survivorship function is a statement of the number of persons out of an initial population of defined size, e.g., 100,000 live births, who would survive or remain free of a defined endpoint condition to age x under the age-specific rates for the specified year. The value of l_{40}, for example, is determined by the cumulative operation of the specific death rates for all ages below 40.

LIFETIME RISK The risk to an individual that a given health effect will occur at any time after exposure without regard for the time at which that effect occurs.

LIKELIHOOD FUNCTION A function constructed from a statistical model and a set of observed data, which gives the probability of the observed data for various values of the unknown model parameters. The parameter values that maximize the probability are the maximum likelihood estimates of the parameters.

LIKELIHOOD RATIO TEST A statistical test based on the ratio of the maximum value of the likelihood function under one statistical model to the maximum value under another statistical model; the models differ in that one includes and the other excludes one or more parameters.

LIKERT SCALE An ordinal scale of responses to a question or statement ordered in a hierarchical sequence, such as from "strongly agree" through "no opinion" to "strongly disagree." Rensis Likert, a social psychologist, developed an empirical method for assigning numerical scores to such a scale.

LINEAR MODEL A statistical model in which the value of a parameter for a given value of a factor, x, is assumed to be equal to $a + bx$, where a and b are constants.

LINEAR REGRESSION Regression analysis of data using linear models.

LINKAGE See GENETIC LINKAGE; RECORD LINKAGE.

LIVE BIRTH WHO definition adopted by Third World Health Assembly, 1950: Live birth is the complete expulsion or extraction from its mother of a product of conception, irrespective of the duration of the pregnancy, which, after such separation, breathes or shows any other evidence of life, such as beating of the heart, pulsation of the umbilical cord, or definite movement of voluntary muscles, whether or not the umbilical cord has been cut or the placenta is attached; each product of such a birth is considered live born.

In the *Report of WHO Expert Committee on Prevention of Perinatal Mortality and Morbidity* (*Technical Report Series* 457, 1970), it is noted that the above definition requires the inclusion as live births of very early and patently nonviable fetuses and that accordingly it is not strictly applied. The committee suggested, therefore, that WHO should introduce a viability criterion into the definition so that very immature fetuses surviving for very short periods were excluded, even though they showed one or more of the transitory signs of life. The Conference for the Tenth Revision of the International Classification of Diseases (*ICD-10*) recommended that the above definitions, adopted for *ICD-9*, should remain unchanged.

LOCUS

1. The position of a point, as defined by the coordinates on a graph.
2. The position that a gene occupies on a chromosome.

LOD SCORE In genetics, the log odds ratio of observed to expected distribution of genetic markers.

LOGIC The branch of philosophy and science that deals with canons of thought and criteria of validity in reasoning. Logic relies on precise definition of tangible objects, terms, and concepts; rational classification; application of fundamental principles of the underlying field of scholarship (mathematics, physics, ethics, etc.); and minimum use of axioms and assumptions. Properly done, epidemiology applies logic to arrive at conclusions about cause-and-effect relationships.[1]

[1] Buck C. Popper's philosophy for epidemiologists. *Int J Epidemiol* 1975; 4:159–168. (See also correspondence and comments in subsequent issues of *Int J Epidemiol*.)

LOGISTIC MODEL A statistical model of an individual's risk (probability of disease y) as a function of a risk factor x:

$$P(y|x) = \frac{1}{1 + e^{-\alpha - \beta x}}$$

where e is the (natural) exponential function. This model has a desirable range, 0 to 1, and other attractive statistical features. In the multiple logistic model, the term βx is replaced by a linear term involving several factors, e.g., $\beta_1 x_1 + \beta_2 x_2$ if there are two factors x_1 and x_2.

LOGIT (Syn: log-odds) The logarithm of the ratio of frequencies of two different categorical outcomes, such as healthy versus sick.

LOGIT MODEL A linear model for the logit (natural log of the odds) of disease as a function of a quantitative factor X:

$$\text{Logit (disease given } X = x) = \alpha + \beta x$$

This model is mathematically equivalent to the LOGISTIC MODEL.

LOG-LINEAR MODEL A statistical model that uses an ANALYSIS OF VARIANCE type of approach for the modeling of frequency counts in contingency tables.

LOG-NORMAL DISTRIBUTION If a variable Y is such that $X = \log Y$ is normally distributed, it is said to have log-normal distribution. This is a SKEW DISTRIBUTION. See also NORMAL DISTRIBUTION.

LONGITUDINAL STUDY See COHORT STUDY.

LOST TO FOLLOW-UP Study subject(s) who cannot or do not complete participation in a study for whatever reason. See also CENSORING.

LOW BIRTH WEIGHT See BIRTH WEIGHT.

"LUMPING AND SPLITTING" Derisive term describing the propensity of epidemiologists to group related phenomena or to separate phenomena that hitherto have been grouped. Epidemiologists are sometimes called "lumpers and splitters."

M

MACHINE LANGUAGE The binary instruction code used by a computer.

MALARIA ENDEMICITY Certain terms used to describe the occurrence of malaria, based on enlarged spleen rates are categorized by WHO as follows:
1. Hypoendemic: Spleen rate in children 2–9 years < 10%.
2. Mesoendemic: Spleen rate 11–50%.
3. Hyperendemic: Spleen rate in children over 50%, in adults usually over 25%.
4. Holoendemic: Spleen rate in children constantly over 75%, adult rate low.

MALARIA PERIODICITY Recurrence at regular intervals of symptoms; periodicity may be quotidian, tertian, or quartan, according to the interval between paroxysms:
1. Quartan: Recurring every third day, i.e., day 1, day 4, day 7, etc.
2. Quotidian: Recurring daily.
3. Tertian: Recurring every alternate day, i.e., day 1, day 3 etc.

MALARIA PATENT PERIOD Period during which parasites are present in peripheral blood.

MALARIA REPRODUCTION RATE Estimated number of malarial infections potentially distributed by the average nonimmune infected individual in a community where neither persons nor mosquitoes were previously infected. See also BASIC REPRODUCTIVE RATE.

MALARIA SURVEY Investigation in selected age-group samples in randomly selected localities to assess malaria endemicity; uses spleen and/or parasite rates as measure of endemicity.

MANN–WHITNEY TEST A test that compares two groups of ordinal scores, showing the probability that they form parts of the same distribution. It is a nonparametric equivalent of the *t*-test.

MANTEL-HAENSZEL ESTIMATE, MANTEL-HAENSZEL ODDS RATIO Mantel and Haenszel[1] provided an adjusted ODDS RATIO as an estimate of relative risk that may be derived from grouped and matched sets of data. It is now known as the Mantel-Haenszel estimate, one of the few eponymous terms of modern epidemiology.

The statistic may be regarded as a type of weighted average of the individual odds ratios, derived from stratifying a sample into a series of strata that are internally homogeneous with respect to confounding factors.

The Mantel-Haenszel summarization method can also be extended to the summarization of rate ratios and rate differences from follow-up studies.

[1] Mantel N. Haenszel W. Statistical aspects of the analysis of data from retrospective studies of disease. *J Natl Cancer Inst* 1959; 22:719–748.

MANTEL-HAENSZEL TEST A summary CHI-SQUARE TEST developed by Mantel and Haenszel for stratified data and used when controlling for CONFOUNDING.

MANTEL'S TREND TEST A regression test of the ODDS RATIO against a numerical variable representing ordered categories of exposure. It can be used to analyze results of a CASE CONTROL STUDY.

MARGIN OF SAFETY An estimate of the ratio of the no-observed-effect level (NOEL) to the level accepted in regulations.

MARGINALS The row and column totals of a contingency table.

MARKOV PROCESS A stochastic process such that the conditional probability distribution for the state at any future instant, given the present state, is unaffected by any additional knowledge of the past history of the system.

MASKED STUDY See BLIND(ED) STUDY.

MASKING (Syn: blinding) Procedure(s) intended to keep participant(s) in a study from knowing some fact(s) or observation(s) that might bias or influence their actions or decisions regarding the study.

MASS ACTION PRINCIPLE A fundamental principle of epidemic theory[1,2]: the incidence of an infectious disease, one SERIAL INTERVAL in the future is dependent on the product of the current prevalence and the number of susceptibles in the population:

$$C_{t+1} = C_t \times S_t \times r$$

where

C_{t+1} = the number of new cases one serial interval in the future
C_t = the number of current cases
S_t = the number of susceptibles
r = the INFECTION TRANSMISSION PARAMETER

[1] Hamer W. Epidemic disease in England. *Lancet* 1906; 1:733–739.
[2] Fine PEM. Herd immunity: History, theory, practice. *Epidemiol Rev* 1993; 15:265–302.

MATCHED CONTROLS See CONTROLS, MATCHED.

MATCHING The process of making a study group and a comparison group comparable with respect to extraneous factors. Several kinds of matching can be distinguished:

Caliper matching is the process of matching comparison group subjects to study group subjects within a specified distance for a continuous variable (e.g., matching age to within 2 years).

Frequency matching requires that the frequency distributions of the matched variable(s) be similar in study and comparison groups.

Category matching is the process of matching study and control group subjects in broad classes such as relatively wide age ranges or occupational groups.

Individual matching relies on identifying individual subjects for comparison, each resembling a study subject on the matched variable(s).

Pair matching is individual matching in which study and comparison subjects are paired.

MATERNAL MORTALITY Several definitions related to maternal mortality have been agreed upon by internationally representative groups under the auspices of the WHO. A *maternal death* is death of a woman while pregnant or within 42 days of termination of pregnancy, irrespective of the duration and the site of pregnancy, from any cause related to or aggravated by the pregnancy or its management but not from accidental or incidental causes. A *late maternal death* is the death of a woman from direct or indirect obstetric causes more than 42 days but less than 1 year after termination of pregnancy. A *pregnancy-related death* is death of a woman while pregnant or within 42 days of termination of pregnancy, irrespective of the cause of death. *Direct obstetric deaths* are those resulting from obstetric complications of the pregnant state (pregnancy, labor, and the puerperium) from interventions, omissions, incorrect treatment, or a chain of events resulting from any of the above.

Indirect obstetric deaths are those resulting from previous existing disease that developed during pregnancy and not due to direct obstetric causes but aggravated by the physiologic effects of pregnancy. In order to improve the quality of maternal mortality data and provide alternative methods of collecting data on deaths during pregnancy or related to it, as well as to encourage the recording of deaths from obstetric causes occurring more than 42 days following termination of pregnancy, the Forty-third World Health Assembly in 1990 adopted the recommendation that countries consider the inclusion on death certificates of questions regarding current pregnancy and pregnancy within 1 year preceding death.

MATERNAL MORTALITY (RATE) The risk of dying from causes associated with childbirth. The numerator is the deaths arising during pregnancy or from puerperal causes, i.e., deaths occurring during and/or due to deliveries, complications of pregnancy, childbirth, and the puerperium. Women exposed to the risk of dying from puerperal causes are those who have been pregnant during the period. Their number being unknown, the number of life births is used as the conventional denominator for computing comparable maternal mortality rates. The formula is

$$\text{Annual maternal mortality rate} = \frac{\substack{\text{Number of deaths from puerperal}\\ \text{causes in a given geographic area}\\ \text{during a given year}}}{\substack{\text{Number of live births that}\\ \text{occurred among the population of}\\ \text{the given geographic area during}\\ \text{the same year}}} \times 1000 \text{ (or 100,000)}$$

There is variation in the duration of the postpartum period in which death may occur and be certified due to "puerperal causes," i.e., "maternal mortality." According to the WHO, a maternal death is defined as the death of a woman while pregnant or within 42 days of termination of pregnancy, irrespective of the duration and the site of pregnancy, from any cause related to or aggravated by the pregnancy or its management but not from accidental or incidental causes.

Maternal deaths should be subdivided into two groups: (1) direct obstetric deaths, resulting from obstetric complications of the pregnant state, and (2) indirect obstetric deaths, resulting from preexisting disease or conditions not due to direct obstetric causes.

Although the WHO defines maternal mortality as death during pregnancy or within 42 days of delivery, in some jurisdictions, a period as long as a year is used.

MATHEMATICAL MODEL A representation of a system, process, or relationship in mathematical form in which equations are used to simulate the behavior of the system or process under study. The model usually consists of two parts: the mathematical structure itself, e.g., Newton's inverse square law or Gauss's "normal" law, and the particular constants or parameters associated with them, such as Newton's gravitational constant or the Gaussian standard deviation.

A mathematical model is deterministic if the relations between the variables involved take on values not allowing for any play of chance. A model is said to be statistical, stochastic, or random if random variation is allowed to enter the picture. See also MODEL.

MAXIMUM ALLOWABLE CONCENTRATION (MAC) See SAFETY STANDARDS.

MAXIMUM LIKELIHOOD ESTIMATE The value for an unknown parameter that maximizes the probability of obtaining exactly the data that were observed.

McNemar's test A form of the CHI-SQUARE TEST for matched-pairs data. It is a special case of the MANTEL-HAENSZEL TEST.

MEAN, ARITHMETIC A MEASURE OF CENTRAL TENDENCY. It is computed by adding all the individual values in the group and dividing by the number of values in the group.

MEAN, GEOMETRIC A MEASURE OF CENTRAL TENDENCY. This is calculated by adding the logarithms of the individual values, calculating their arithmetic mean, and converting back by taking the antilogarithm. Can be calculated only for positive values.

MEAN, HARMONIC A MEASURE OF CENTRAL TENDENCY computed by summing the reciprocals of all the individual values and dividing the resulting sum into the number of values.

MEASURE OF ASSOCIATION A quantity that expresses the strength of association between variables. Commonly used measures of association are differences between means, proportions or rates, the rate ratio, the odds ratio, and correlation and regression coefficients.

MEASUREMENT The procedure of applying a standard scale to a variable or to a set of values.

MEASUREMENT BIAS Systematic error arising from inaccurate measurements (or classification) of subjects on study variable(s).

MEASUREMENT SCALE The range of possible values for a measurement (e.g., the set of possible responses to a question, the physically possible range for a set of body weights). Measurement scales can be classified according to the quantitative character of the scale:

1. *Dichotomous scale:* One that arranges items into either of two mutually exclusive categories.
2. *Nominal scale:* Classification into unordered qualitative categories; e.g., race, religion, and country of birth as measurements of individual attributes are purely nominal scales, as there is no inherent order to their categories.
3. *Ordinal scale:* Classification into ordered qualitative categories, e.g., social class (I, II, III, etc.), where the values have a distinct order, but their categories are qualitative in that there is no natural (numerical) distance between their possible values.
4. *Interval scale:* An (equal) interval involves assignment of values with a natural distance between them, so that a particular distance (interval) between two values in one region of the scale meaningfully represents the same distance between two values in another region of the scale. Examples include Celsius and Fahrenheit temperature, date of birth.
5. *Ratio scale:* A ratio is an interval scale with a true zero point, so that ratios between values are meaningfully defined. Examples are absolute temperature, weight, height, blood count, and income, as in each case it is meaningful to speak of one value as being so many times greater or less than another value.

MEASUREMENT, TERMINOLOGY OF There is sometimes uncertainty about the terms used to describe the properties of measurement: *accuracy, precision, validity, reliability, repeatability,* and *reproducibility. Accuracy* and *precision* are often used synonymously, *validity* is defined variously, and *reliability, repeatability,* and *reproducibility* are often used interchangeably.

Etymologies are helpful in making a case for preferred usages, but they are not always decisive. *Accuracy* is from the Latin *cura* (care), and while this may be of interest to those in the health field, it does not illuminate the origins of the standard definition, that is, "conforming to a standard or a true value" *(OED). Accuracy* is distinguished from *precision* in this way: A measurement or statement can reflect or represent a true value without detail. A temperature reading of 37.5°C is accurate, but it is not precise if a more refined thermometer registers a temperature of 37.543°C.

Precision (from Latin *praecidere,* cut short) is the quality of being sharply defined through exact detail. A faulty measurement may be expressed precisely but may not be accurate. Measurements should be both accurate and precise, but the two terms are not synonymous. *Consistency* or *reliability* describes the property of measurements or results that conform to themselves.

Reliability (Latin *religare,* to bind) is defined by the *OED* as a quality that is sound and dependable. Its epidemiologic usage is similar; a result or measurement is said to be reliable when it is stable, i.e., when repetition of an experiment or measurement gives the same results. The terms *repeatability* and *reproducibility* are synonymous (the *OED* defines each in terms of the other), but they do not refer to a quality of measurement, rather only to the action of performing something more than once. Thus, a way of discovering whether or not a measurement is reliable is to repeat or reproduce it. The terms *repeatability* and *reproducibility,* formed from their respective verbs, are used inaccurately when they are substituted for *reliability,* a noun that refers to the measuring procedure rather than the attribute being measured. However, in common usage, both repeatability and reproducibility refer to the capacity of a measuring procedure to produce the same result on each occasion in a series of procedures conducted under identical conditions.

Validity is used correctly when it agrees with the standard definition given by the *OED:* "sound and sufficient." If, in the epidemiologic sense, a test measures what it purports to measure (it is sufficient) then the test is said to be valid. See also ACCURACY; PRECISION; RELIABILITY; REPEATABILITY; VALIDITY.

MEASURE OF CENTRAL TENDENCY A general term for several characteristics of the distribution of a set of values or measurements around a value or values at or near the middle of the set. The principal measures of central tendency are the MEAN (average), MEDIAN, and MODE.

MECHANICAL TRANSMISSION Transmission of pathogens by a vector (e.g., a housefly) without biological development in or dependence on the vector. Many fecal-oral infections are spread by this means. See also VECTOR-BORNE INFECTION.

MEDIAN A MEASURE OF CENTRAL TENDENCY. The simplest division of a set of measurements is into two parts—the lower and the upper half. The point on the scale that divides the group in this way is called the "median."

MEDIATOR (MEDIATING) VARIABLE See INTERMEDIATE VARIABLE.

MEDICAL AUDIT A health service evaluation procedure in which selected data from patients' charts are summarized in tables displaying such data as average length of stay or duration of an episode of care, the frequency of diagnostic and therapeutic procedures, and outcomes of care arranged by diagnostic category. These are often compared with predetermined norms.

MEDICAL CARE See HEALTH CARE.

MEDICAL RECORD A file of information relating to transaction(s) in personal health care. In addition to facts about a patient's illness, medical records nearly always contain other information. The information in medical records includes the following:

1. Clinical, i.e., diagnosis, treatment, progress, etc.
2. Demographic, i.e., age, sex, birthplace, residence, etc.
3. Sociocultural, i.e., language, ethnic origin, religion, etc.

4. Sociological, i.e., family (next of kin), occupation, etc.
5. Economic, i.e., method of payment (fee-for-service, indigent, etc.).
6. Administrative, i.e., site of care, provider, etc.
7. "Behavioral," e.g., record of broken appointment may indicate dissatisfaction with service provided.

MEDICAL STATISTICS See BIOSTATISTICS.

MENDEL'S LAWS Derived from the pioneering genetic studies of Gregor Mendel (1822–1884). Mendel's first law states that genes are particulate units that segregate; i.e., members of the same pair of genes are never present in the same gamete, but always separate and pass to different gametes. Mendel's second law states that genes assort independently; i.e., members of different pairs of genes move to gametes independently of one another.

METAANALYSIS The process of using statistical methods to combine the results of different studies. In the biomedical sciences, the systematic, organized and structured evaluation of a problem of interest, using information (commonly in the form of statistical tables or other data) from a number of independent studies of the problem. A frequent application has been the pooling of results from a set of randomized controlled trials, none in itself necessarily powerful enough to demonstrate statistically significant differences, but in aggregate, capable of so doing. Metaanalysis has a qualitative component, i.e., application of predetermined criteria of quality (e.g., completeness of data, absence of biases), and a quantitative component, i.e., integration of the numerical information. Statistical analysis of a collection of analyzed results, sometimes of raw data from individual studies, usually previously published peer-reviewed studies. The aim is to integrate the findings, pool the data, and identify the overall trend of results.[1] An essential prerequisite is that the studies must stand up to critical appraisal, and various biases, e.g., PUBLICATION BIAS, must be allowed for.[2]

[1] Dickerson K, Berlin JA. Meta-analysis: State of the science. *Epidemiol Rev* 1992; 14:154–176.
[2] Petitti DB. *Meta-Analysis, Decision Analysis and Cost-Effectiveness Analysis: Methods for Quantitative Synthesis in Medicine.* New York: Oxford University Press, 1994.

METHODOLOGY The scientific study of methods. Methodology should not be confused with methods. The word *methodology* is all too often used when the writer means *method*.

MIASMA THEORY An explanation for the origin of epidemics, the "miasma theory" was implied by many ancient writers, and made explicit by Lancisi in *De noxiis paludum effluviis* (1717). It was based on the notion that when the air was of a "bad quality" (a state that was not precisely defined, but that was supposedly due to decaying organic matter), the persons breathing that air would become ill. Malaria ("bad air") is the classic example of a disease that was long attributed to miasmata. "Miasma" was believed to pass from cases to susceptibles in these diseases considered contagious.

MIGRANT STUDIES Studies taking advantage of migration to one country by those from other countries with different physical and biological environments, cultural background and/or genetic makeup, and different morbidity or mortality experience. Comparisons are made between the mortality or morbidity experience of the migrant groups with that of their current country of residence and/or their country of origin. Sometimes the experiences of a number of different groups who have migrated to the same country have been compared.

MILL'S CANONS In *A System of Logic* (1856), J. S. Mill devised logical strategies (canons) from which causal relationships may be inferred. Four in particular are pertinent to epidemiology: the methods of agreement, difference, residues, and concomitant variation.

Method of agreement (first canon): "If two or more instances of the phenomenon under investigation have only one circumstance in common, the circumstance in which alone all the instances agree, is the cause (or effect) of the given phenomenon."

Method of difference (second canon): "If an instance in which the phenomenon under investigation occurs, and an instance in which it does not occur, have every circumstance in common save one, that one occurring only in the former, the circumstance in which alone the two instances differ is the effect, or cause or a necessary part of the cause, of the phenomenon."

Method of residues (fourth canon): "Subduct from any phenomenon such part as is known by previous inductions to be the effect of certain antecedents, and the residue of the phenomenon is the effect of the remaining antecedents."

Method of concomitant variation (fifth canon): "Whatever phenomenon varies in any manner whether another phenomenon varies in some particular manner, is either a cause or an effect of that phenomenon, or is connected with it through some fact of causation."

MINIMUM DATA SET (Syn: uniform basic data set) A widely agreed upon and generally accepted set of terms and definitions constituting a core of data acquired for medical records and employed for developing statistics suitable for diverse types of analyses and users. Such sets have been developed for birth and death certificates, ambulatory care, hospital care, and long-term care. See also BIRTH CERTIFICATE; DEATH CERTIFICATE; HOSPITAL DISCHARGE ABSTRACT SYSTEM.

MISCLASSIFICATION The erroneous classification of an individual, a value, or an attribute into a category other than that to which it should be assigned. The probability of misclassification may be the same in all study groups (nondifferential misclassification) or may vary between groups (differential misclassification).

MISSION The purpose for which an organization exists. See also GOAL, OBJECTIVE, TARGET.

MOBILITY, GEOGRAPHIC Movement of persons from one permanent place of residence (country or region) to another.

MOBILITY, SOCIAL Movement from one defined socioeconomic group to another, either upward or downward. Downward social mobility, which can be related to impaired health (e.g., alcoholism, schizophrenia, or mental retardation), is sometimes referred to as "social drift."

MODE One of the MEASURES OF CENTRAL TENDENCY. The most frequently occurring value in a set of observations.

MODEL

1. An abstract representation of the relationship between logical, analytical, or empirical components of a system. See also MATHEMATICAL MODEL.
2. A formalized expression of a theory or the causal situation that is regarded as having generated observed data.
3. (Animal) model: an experimental system that uses animals, because humans cannot be used for ethical or other reasons.
4. A small-scale simulation, e.g., by using an "average region" with characteristics resembling those of the whole country.

In epidemiology, the use of models began with an effort to predict the onset and course of epidemics. In the second report of the Registrar-General of England and

Wales (1840), William Farr developed the beginnings of a predictive model for communicable disease epidemics. He had recognized regularities in the smallpox epidemics of the 1830s. By calculating frequency curves for these past outbreaks, he estimated the deaths to be expected. See also DEMONSTRATION MODEL; MATHE-MATICAL MODEL; THEORETICAL EPIDEMIOLOGY.

MODEM An electronic device that encodes computerized information in a form suitable for transmission through a telephone circuit.

MODERATOR VARIABLE (Syn: qualifier variable) In a study of a possible causal factor and an outcome, a moderator variable is a third variable exhibiting statistical inter-action by virtue of its being antecedent or intermediate in the causal process under study. If it is antecedent, it is termed a conditional moderator variable or EFFECT MODIFIER; if it is intermediate, it is a contingent moderator variable. See also INTER-ACTION; INTERMEDIATE VARIABLE.

MOLECULAR EPIDEMIOLOGY The use in epidemiologic studies of techniques of molecu-lar biology.[1] Techniques such as DNA typing are used to detect, identify, and mea-sure distinct molecular structures, which may be normal, variant, or damaged by disease or environmental exposures. The measures may refer to exposure, early biological response, host characteristics that influence response (susceptibility) or other mediating biological events. Techniques of molecular epidemiology have been used to identify precisely the genotype of pathogenic microorganisms and so to trace the pathway taken by a specific strain in infecting a group of people. Viral DNA can be measured in host cells and their genome. Molecular techniques are used in cancer epidemiology to identify, characterize, and measure molecular changes involved in carcinogenesis (xenobiotic DNA adducts, somatic genetic muta-tions); heritable genetic polymorphism relevant to metabolic susceptibility; and "cancer family" genes. There is debate about the use of the term *molecular epidemiol-ogy*[2]—it is really a level and method of measurement rather than a discipline with substantive research content. Nonetheless, it has made many valuable contributions to biomedical and clinical science and has great promise for the future.

[1] Schulte PA, Perera FP: *Molecular Epidemiology; Principles and Practices*. Orlando, FL: Academic Press, 1993.
[2] McMichael AJ: "Molecular epidemiology": New pathway or new travelling companion? *Am J Epi-demiol* 1994; 140:1–11.

MONITORING
1. The performance and analysis of routine measurements, aimed at detecting changes in the environment or health status of populations. Not to be con-fused with SURVEILLANCE. To some, monitoring also implies intervention in the light of observed measurements.
2. Continuous measurement of the effect of an intervention on the health status of a population or environment. Not to be confused with SURVEILLANCE, al-though the techniques of surveillance may be used in monitoring. The process of collecting and analyzing information about the implementation of a pro-gram for the purpose of identifying problems such as noncompliance and taking corrective action. (Source: WHO AIDS Series, No. 5; Geneva: WHO, 1989.)
3. In management, the continuous oversight of the implementation of an activ-ity, seeking to ensure that input deliveries, work schedules, targeted outputs, and other required actions are proceeding according to plan.

MONOTONIC SEQUENCE A sequence is said to be monotonic increasing if each value is greater than or equal to the previous one, and monotonic decreasing if each value is less than or equal to the previous one. If equality of values is excluded, we speak of a strictly (increasing or decreasing) monotonic sequence.

MONTE CARLO STUDY, TRIAL Complex relationships that are difficult to solve by mathematical analysis are sometimes studied by computer experiments that simulate and analyze a sequence of events, using random numbers. Such experiments are called Monte Carlo trials or studies in recognition of Monte Carlo as one of the gambling capitals of the world.

MORBIDITY Any departure, subjective or objective, from a state of physiological or psychological well-being. In this sense *sickness, illness,* and *morbid condition* are similarly defined and synonymous (but see DISEASE).

The WHO Expert Committee on Health Statistics noted in its Sixth report (1959) that morbidity could be measured in terms of three units: (1) persons who were ill; (2) the illnesses (periods or spells of illness) that these persons experienced; and (3) the duration (days, weeks, etc.) of these illnesses. See also HEALTH INDEX; INCIDENCE RATE; NOTIFIABLE DISEASE; PREVALENCE RATE.

MORBIDITY RATE A term, preferably avoided, used indiscriminately to refer to incidence or prevalence rates of disease.

MORBIDITY SURVEY A method for estimating the prevalence and/or incidence of disease or diseases in a population. A morbidity survey is usually designed simply to ascertain the facts as to disease distribution and not to test a hypothesis. See also CROSS-SECTIONAL STUDY; HEALTH SURVEY.

MORTALITY RATE See DEATH RATE.

MORTALITY STATISTICS Statistical tables compiled from the information contained in DEATH CERTIFICATES. Most administrative jurisdictions in all nations produce tables of mortality statistics. These may be published at regular intervals; they usually show numbers of deaths and/or rates by age, sex, cause, and sometimes other variables.

MOVING AVERAGES (Syn: rolling averages) A method of smoothing irregularities in trend data, such as long-term secular trends in incidence or mortality rates. Graphical display of 3- or 5-year moving averages makes it easier to discern long-term trends in rates that otherwise might be obscured by short-term fluctuations.

MULTICOLLINEARITY In multiple regression analysis, a situation in which at least some of the independent variables are highly correlated with each other. Such a situation can result in inaccurate estimates of the parameters in the regression model.

MULTIFACTORIAL ETIOLOGY See MULTIPLE CAUSATION.

MULTILEVEL ANALYSIS Methods of analysis that explain individual outcomes in terms of both individual and environmental or aggregate variables, thus avoiding the ECO-LOGIC FALLACY.[1]

[1] Von Korff M, Koepsell T, Curry S, Diehr P. Multilevel analysis in epidemiologic research on health behaviors and outcomes. *Am J Epidemiol* 1992; 135:1077–1082.

MULTINOMIAL DISTRIBUTION The probability distribution associated with the classification of each of a sample of individuals into one of several mutually exclusive and exhaustive categories. When the number of categories is two, the distribution is called binomial. See also BINOMIAL DISTRIBUTION.

MULTIPHASE SAMPLING Method of sampling that gathers some information from a large sample and more detailed information from subsamples within this sample, either at the same time or later.

MULTIPHASIC SCREENING See SCREENING.

MULTIPLE CAUSATION (Syn: multifactorial etiology) This term is used to refer to the concept that a given disease or other outcome may have more than one cause. A combination of causes or alternative combinations of causes may be required to produce the effect.

MULTIPLE COMPARISON TECHNIQUES Statistical procedures to adjust for differences in probability levels when setting up simultaneous confidence limits in several distributions or sets of data or to compare the means of several groups. *Tukey's method* is the most conservative; this uses the difference between the largest and smallest means as a measure of their dispersion; the q statistic, based on the α level, and the number of groups are used as multipliers of the standard deviation. The *Bonferroni correction* adjusts the α error level to compensate for multiple comparisons between three or more groups or two or more response variables.

MULTIPLE LOGISTIC MODEL See LOGISTIC MODEL.

MULTIPLE OF THE MEDIAN A simple method of standardization that allows adjustment for variables such as age and sex, is directly proportional to the magnitude of the original measurements, and is not much affected by variation in measurement errors. However, the method is criticized because the multiple of the median is affected by the distribution of results used to determine the median, and there is no correction for the spread of the data. For these reasons the z SCORE is preferable.

MULTIPLE REGRESSION TECHNIQUES Varieties of multiple regression analysis used in epidemiology include linear regression analysis, using a linear regression model, and logistic regression analysis, which uses a multiple logistic regression model. Details can be found in monographs on biostatistics.

MULTIPLE RISK Where more than one risk factor for the development of a disease or other outcome is present, and their combined presence results in an increased risk, we speak of "multiple risk." The increased risk may be due to the additive effects of the risks associated with the separate risk factors, or to SYNERGISM.

MULTIPLICATIVE MODEL A model in which the joint effect of two or more causes is the product of their effects. For instance, if factor a multiplies risk by the amount a in the absence of factor b, and factor b multiplies risk by the amount b in the absence of factor a, the combined effect of factors a and b on risk is $a \times b$. See also ADDITIVE MODEL.

MULTISTAGE MODEL A mathematical model, mainly for carcinogenesis, based on the theory that a specific carcinogen may affect one of a number of stages in the development of cancer.

MULTIVARIATE ANALYSIS A set of techniques used when the variation in several variables has to be studied simultaneously. In statistics, any analytic method that allows the simultaneous study of two or more DEPENDENT VARIABLES.

MUTATION Heritable change in the genetic material not caused by genetic segregation or recombination that is transmitted to daughter cells and to succeeding generations provided it is not a dominant lethal factor.

MUTATION RATE The frequency with which mutations occur per gene or per generation.

N

NATIONAL DEATH INDEX A computerized central registry of deaths in the United States, started in 1979 and operated by the U.S. National Center for Health Statistics, that facilitates mortality followup; cf. CANADIAN MORTALITY DATABASE.

NATURAL EXPERIMENT Naturally occurring circumstances in which subsets of the population have different levels of exposure to a supposed causal factor, in a situation resembling an actual experiment where human subjects would be randomly allocated to groups. The presence of persons in a particular group is nonrandom. The term derives from the work of John Snow (1813–1858), who investigated the distribution of cholera cases in London in relation to the source of their water supply. It would have been unethical for Snow to allocate subjects to groups exposed to a lethal infection, but tracing the source of their drinking water, using SHOE-LEATHER EPIDEMIOLOGY, gave him the opportunity to make crucially important observations.

To turn this grand experiment to account, all that was required was to learn the supply of water to each individual house where a fatal attack of cholera might occur . . . I resolved to spare no exertion which might be necessary to ascertain the exact effect of the water supply on the progress of the epidemic, in the places where all the circumstances were so happily adapted for the inquiry . . . I had no reason to doubt the correctness of the conclusions I had drawn from the great number of facts already in my possession, but I felt that the circumstances of the cholera-poisoning passing down the sewers into a great river, and being distributed through miles of pipes, and yet producing its specific effects was a fact of so startling a nature, and of so vast importance to the community, that it could not be too rigidly examined or established on too firm a basis. (Snow, J. *On the Mode of Communication of Cholera,* London, 1855)

Another example is the reduction in death rates from smoking-related causes among doctors, contrasted with other professional men of comparable age, that followed their cessation of smoking some years earlier than other men.

NATURAL HISTORY OF DISEASE The course of a disease from onset (inception) to resolution. Many diseases have certain well-defined stages that, taken all together, are referred to as the "natural history of the disease" in question. These stages are as follows:

1. Stage of pathological onset.
2. Presymptomatic stage: from onset to the first appearance of symptoms and/or signs. SCREENING tests may lead to earlier detection.
3. Clinically manifest disease, which may progress inexorably to a fatal termination, be subject to remissions and relapses, or regress spontaneously, leading to recovery.

Some diseases have precursors; for example, elevated serum cholesterol is among the precursors of coronary heart disease. Precursors may long precede the stage of pathologic onset, and some—e.g., elevated serum cholesterol—can be detected by screening-level tests. Other conditions may be preceded by genetically determined predisposition. Early detection, as by screening, and intervention can alter the natural history of many diseases, especially cardiovascular disease and cancer. The term has also been used to mean "descriptive epidemiology of disease."

NATURAL HISTORY STUDY A study, generally longitudinal, designed to yield information about the natural course of a disease or condition.

NATURAL RATE OF INCREASE (DECREASE) See GROWTH RATE OF POPULATION.

NEAREST NEIGHBOR METHOD A means of analyzing the spatial patterns of a free-living population. A term from veterinary epidemiology. Random sampling points are located throughout an area and the distance from each point to the nearest individual is measured; alternatively, individuals are selected at random and from each of these the distance to the nearest neighbor is measured.

NECESSARY CAUSE A causal factor whose presence is required for the occurrence of the effect and whose presence is always followed by the effect. See also ASSOCIATION; CAUSALITY.

NEEDLE STICK Puncture of the skin by a needle that may have been contaminated by contact with an infected patient. See also SHARPS.

NEEDS (Syn: health needs, perceived needs, professionally defined needs, unmet needs) This term has both a precise and an all-but-indefinable meaning in the context of public health. We speak of needs in precise numerical terms when we refer to specific indicators of disease or premature death that require intervention because their level is above that generally accepted in the society or community in question. For example, an infant mortality rate two or three times greater than the national average in a particular community is an indicator of unmet health needs of infants in that community (not to be confused with a need for more or better medical care). It should be clear that even in this seemingly precise usage, there are implied value judgments. It must be explicitly stated that "needs" always reflect prevailing value judgments as well as the existing ability to control a particular public health problem. Thus, sputum-positive pulmonary tuberculosis was not recognized as a health need in 1850 but was by 1900 in the industrialized nations; the ill effects of cigarette smoking must now be universally acknowledged as a health need; and child abuse is increasingly regarded as a public health problem, to which we could apply the term *professionally defined need*.

(See Vickers GR. What sets the goals of public health? *Lancet* 1:599, 1958.)

NEONATAL MORTALITY RATE

1. In VITAL STATISTICS, the number of deaths in infants under 28 days of age in a given period, usually a year, per 1000 live births in that period.
2. In obstetric and perinatal research, the term *neonatal mortality rate* is often used to denote the cumulative MORTALITY RATE of live-born infants within 28 days of age.

NESTED CASE CONTROL STUDY A case control study in which cases and controls are drawn from the population in a COHORT STUDY. As some data are already available about both cases and controls, the effects of some potential confounding variables are reduced or eliminated. In this type of case control study, a set of controls is selected from subjects at risk at the time of occurrence of each case that arises in a cohort, thus allowing for the confounding effect of time in the analysis.[1]

---

[1] Wacholder S, McLaughlin JK, Silverman DT, Mandel JS: Selection of controls in case-control studies. I. Principles. *Am J Epidemiol* 1992; 135:1019–1028;
Wacholder S, Silverman DT, McLaughlin JK, Mandel JS: Selection of controls in case-control studies. II. Types of controls. *Am J Epidemiol* 1992; 135–1029–1041.
————JS: Selection of controls in case-control studies. III. Design options. *Am J Epidemiol* 1992; 135:1042–1050.

NET MIGRATION The numerical difference between immigration and emigration.

NET MIGRATION RATE The net effect of immigration and emigration on an area's population expressed as an increase or decrease per 1000 population of the area in a given year.

NET REPRODUCTION RATE (NRR) The average number of female children born per woman in a cohort subject to a given set of age-specific fertility rates, a given set of age-specific mortality rates, and a given sex ratio at birth. This rate measures replacement fertility under given conditions of fertility and mortality: it is the ratio of daughters to mothers assuming continuation of the specified conditions of fertility and mortality. It is a measure of population growth from one generation to another under constant conditions. This rate is similar to the gross reproduction rate, but takes into account that some women will die before completing their childbearing years. An NRR of 1.00 means that each generation of mothers is having exactly enough daughters to replace itself in the population. See also GROSS REPRODUCTION RATE.

NET REPRODUCTIVE RATE (R) (Syn: case reproduction rate) In infectious disease epidemiology, the average number of secondary cases that will occur in a mixed host population of susceptibles and non-susceptibles when one infected individual is introduced. Its relationship to the BASIC REPRODUCTIVE RATE (R_0) is given by

$$R = R_0 x$$

where x is the proportion of the host population that is susceptible.

NEW YORK STATE IDENTIFICATION AND INTELLIGENCE SYSTEM (NYSIIS) A method of identifying individuals for RECORD LINKAGE based on phonetic spelling of full names, sequence of digits for birthdate, birthplace, sex, name at birth, and parents' names. See also HOGBEN NUMBER; SOUNDEX CODE.

NIDUS A focus of infection. The term can be used to describe any heterogeneity in the distribution of a disease but is usually applied to a small area in which conditions favor occurrence and spread of a communicable disease; also, the site of origin of a pathological process.

NOCEBO An unpleasant effect attributable to administration of a placebo. A jargon term preferably avoided.

NOISE (IN DATA) This term is used when extraneous uncontrolled variables and/or errors influence the distribution of measurements that are made in a study, thus rendering difficult or impossible the determination of relationships between variables under scrutiny.

NOMENCLATURE A list of all approved terms for describing and recording observations.

NOMINAL SCALE See MEASUREMENT SCALE.

NOMOGRAM A form of line chart showing scales for the variables involved in a particular formula in such a way that corresponding values for each variable lie on a straight line intersecting all the scales.

NONCONCURRENT STUDY See HISTORICAL COHORT STUDY.

NONDIFFERENTIAL MISCLASSIFICATION See MISCLASSIFICATION.

NONEXPERIMENTAL STUDY See OBSERVATIONAL STUDY.

NONPARAMETRIC METHODS See DISTRIBUTION-FREE METHOD.

NONPARAMETRIC TEST See DISTRIBUTION-FREE METHOD.

NONPARTICIPANTS (Syn: nonresponders) Members of a study sample or population who do not take part in the study for whatever reason, or members of a target population who do not participate in an activity. Differences between participants and nonparticipants have been demonstrated repeatedly in studies of many kinds, and this is often a source of BIAS.

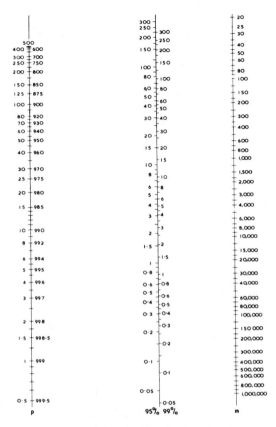

Nomogram of confidence limits to a rate.

From Rosenbaum, Nomograms for rates per 1000, *Br Med J* 1:169–170, 1963.

Nomogram of confidence limits to a rate. With permission.

NO-OBSERVED-EFFECT LEVEL (NOEL) The highest dose at which no adverse health effects are detected in an animal population. A NOEL-SF is a no-observed-effects level with an added safety factor for human exposures, used in setting human safety standards. In practice, the safety factor added is commonly two or more orders of magnitude, i.e., a hundredfold or a thousandfold greater than the NOEL.

N-OF-ONE STUDY (Syn: single-patient trial) A variation of a randomized controlled trial in which a sequence of alternative treatment regimens is randomly allocated to a patient. The outcomes of regimens are compared, with the aim of deciding on the optimum regimen for the patient.[1]

[1]Guyatt G, Sackett D, Taylow DW, et al. Determining optimal therapy—Randomized trials in individual patients. *N Engl J Med* 1986; 314:889–892.

NORM This term has two quite distinct meanings:

1. The first is "what is usual," e.g., the range into which blood pressure values usually fall in a population group, the dietary or infant feeding practices that are usual in a given culture, or the way that a given illness is usually treated in a given health care system.
2. The second sense is "what is desirable," e.g., the range of blood pressures that a given authority regards as being indicative of present good health or as

predisposing to future good health, the dietary or infant feeding practices that are valued in a given culture, or the health care procedures or facilities for health care that a given authority regards as desirable.

In the latter sense, norms may be used as criteria when evaluating health care, in order to determine the degree of conformity with what is desirable, the average length of stay of patients in hospital, etc. A distinction is sometimes made between norms, defined as quantitative indexes based on research, and standards, which are fixed arbitrarily.

NORMAL This term has three distinct meanings. Conceptual difficulties may arise if these different meanings are not specified or if the area of their overlap is not clearly understood.

1. Within the usual range of variation in a given population or population group, or frequently occurring in a given population or group. In this sense, "normal" is frequently defined as, "within a range extending from two standard deviations below the mean to two standard deviations above the mean," or "between specified (e.g., the 10th and 90th) percentiles of the distribution."

2. In good health, indicative or predictive of good health, or conducive to good health. For a diagnostic or screening test, a "normal" result is one in a range within which the probability of a specific disease is low (see also NORMAL LIMITS).

3. (Of a distribution) Gaussian; see also NORMAL DISTRIBUTION.

NORMAL DISTRIBUTION (Syn: Gaussian distribution) The continuous frequency distribution of infinite range represented by the equation

$$f(x) = \frac{1}{(2\pi\sigma^2)^{1/2}} e^{-(x-\mu)^2/2\sigma^2}$$

where x is the abscissa, $f(x)$ is the ordinate, μ is the mean, e is the natural logarithm, 2.718 and σ the standard deviation. All possible values of the variable are displayed on the horizontal axis. The frequency (probability) of each value is displayed on the vertical axis, producing the graph of the normal distribution.

The properties of a normal distribution include the following: (1) It is a continuous, symmetrical distribution; both tails extend to infinity; (2) the arithmetic mean,

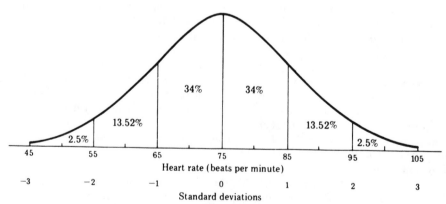

Normal distribution of heart rate. From Rimm AA, Hartz, AJ, Kalbfleish JH, Anderson AJ, Hoffmann RG: *Basic Biostatistics in Medicine and Epidemiology.* New York: Appleton-Century-Crofts, 1980. With permission.

mode, and median are identical; and (3) its shape is completely determined by the mean and standard deviation.

NORMAL LIMITS The limits of the "normal" range of a test or measurement, in the sense of being indicative of or conducive to good health. One way to determine normal limits is to compare the values obtained when the measurements are made in two groups, one that is healthy and has been found to remain healthy, the other ill or subsequently found to become ill. The result may be two overlapping distributions. Outside the area where the distributions overlap, a given value clearly identifies the presence or absence of disease or some other manifestation of poor health. If a value falls into the area of overlap, the individual may belong to either the normal or the abnormal group. The choice of the normal limits depends upon the relative importance attached to the identification of individuals as healthy or unhealthy. See also FALSE NEGATIVE; FALSE POSITIVE; SENSITIVITY AND SPECIFICITY.

NORMATIVE Pertaining to the normal, usual, accepted standard or values. See also NORM.

NOSOCOMIAL Arising while a patient is in a hospital or as a result of being in a hospital; relating to a hospital; denoting a new disorder (unrelated to the patient's primary condition) associated with being in a hospital.

NOSOCOMIAL INFECTION (Syn: hospital-acquired infection) An infection originating in a medical facility, e.g., occurring in a patient in a hospital or other health care facility in whom the infection was not present or incubating at the time of admission. Includes infections acquired in the hospital but appearing after discharge; it also includes such infections among staff.

NOSOGRAPHY, NOSOLOGY Classification of ill persons into groups, whatever the criteria for their classification, and agreement as to the boundaries of the groups, is called "nosology." The assignment of names to each disease entity in the group results in a nomenclature of disease entities, or nosography.[1]

[1] Faber K. *Nosography in Modern Internal Medicine*. New York: Hoeber, 1923.

NOTIFIABLE DISEASE A disease that, by statutory requirements, must be reported to the public health authority in the pertinent jurisdiction when the diagnosis is made.

A disease deemed of sufficient importance to the public health to require that its occurrence be reported to health authorities.

The reporting to public health authorities of communicable diseases is, unfortunately, very incomplete. The reasons for this include diagnostic inexactitude; the desire of patients and physicians to conceal the occurrence of conditions carrying a social stigma, e.g., sexually transmitted diseases; and the indifference of physicians to the usefulness of information about such diseases as hepatitis, influenza, and measles. Yet notifications are extremely important. They provide the starting point for investigations into the failure of preventive measures such as immunizations, for tracing sources of infection, for finding common vehicles of infection, for describing the geographic clustering of infection, and for various other purposes, depending upon the particular disease.

N.S., n.s. Abbreviation, usually written lower case, for not statistically significant.

NULL HYPOTHESIS (Syn: test hypothesis) The statistical hypothesis that one variable has no association with another variable or set of variables, or that two or more population distributions do not differ from one another. In simplest terms, the null hypothesis states that the results observed in a study, experiment, or test are no different from what might have occurred as a result of the operation of chance alone.

NUMBER NEEDED TO TREAT In clinical treatment regimens, the number of patients with a specified condition who must follow the specified regimen for a prescribed period in order to prevent the occurrence of specified complication(s) or adverse outcome(s) of the condition. This number is the reciprocal of the ABSOLUTE RISK reduction, i.e., the difference between the occurrence rates of adverse outcomes in the treated and placebo groups in a clinical trial. In an example given by Sackett et al.,[1] adverse outcomes in the treated and placebo groups respectively are 4% (0.04) and 10% (0.10). This gives an absolute risk reduction of 0.06, and the reciprocal of this is 17; i.e., on average, 17 patients have to be treated in order to prevent one of them from having an adverse outcome.

[1] Sackett DL, Haynes RB, Guyatt GH, Tugwell P: *Clinical Epidemiology: A Basic Science for Clinical Medicine.* Boston: Little, Brown, 1991:205–209.

NUMERATOR The upper portion of a fraction used to calculate a rate or a ratio.

NUMERICAL TAXONOMY The construction of homogeneous groupings or taxa using numerical methods.

O

OBJECTIVE The precisely stated end to which efforts are directed, specifying the population outcome, variable(s) to be measured, etc. See also GOAL, TARGET.

OBSERVATIONAL STUDY (Syn: nonexperimental study) Epidemiologic study that does not involve any intervention, experimental or otherwise. Such a study may be one in which nature is allowed to take its course, with changes in one characteristic being studied in relation to changes in other characteristics. Analytic epidemiologic methods,[1] such as case-control and cohort study designs, are properly called observational epidemiology because the investigator is observing without intervention other than to record, classify, count, and statistically analyze results.

[1] Kelsey JL, Thompson WD, Evans AL. *Methods in Observational Epidemiology.* New York: Oxford University Press, 1986.

OBSERVER BIAS Systematic difference between a true value and that actually observed, due to OBSERVER VARIATION.

OBSERVER VARIATION (ERROR) Variation (or error) due to failure of the observer to measure or to identify a phenomenon accurately. Observer variation erodes scientific credibility whenever it appears. Sir Thomas Browne in *Pseudodoxia Epidemica* (1646), subtitled "Enquiries into very many commonly received tenents and presumed truths," recognized several sources of error: "the common infirmity of human nature, the erroneous disposition of the people, misapprehension, fallacy or false deduction, credulity, obstinate adherence to authority, the belief in popular conceits, the endeavours of Satan."

All observations are subject to variation. Discrepancies between repeated observations by the same observer and between different observers are to be expected; these can be diminished but probably never absolutely eliminated.

Variation may arise from several sources. The observer may miss an abnormality or think he has found one where none is present; a measurement or a test may give incorrect results due to faulty technique or incorrect reading and recording of the results; or the observer may misinterpret the information. Two varieties of observer variation are interobserver variation, i.e., the amount observers vary from one another when reporting on the same material, and intraobserver variation, the amount one observer varies between observations when reporting more than once on the same material.

OCCAM'S RAZOR The principle of scientific parsimony. The 14th-century philosopher William of Occam said: *Essentia non sunt multiplicanda praeter necessitatem;* i.e., assumptions to explain a phenomenon must not be multiplied beyond necessity. In *The Grammar of Science* (1892), Karl Pearson called this the most important canon in the whole field of logical thought. This maxim does not contradict the conclusion that multiple causes may operate in a system. The number of possible causes implicated depends upon the frame of reference of the investigator and the scope of the inquiry.

OCCUPATIONAL HEALTH (Syn: occupational medicine, industrial hygiene) The specialized practice of medicine, public health, and ancillary health professions in an occupational setting. Its aims are to promote health as well as to prevent occupationally related diseases and injuries and the impairments arising therefrom, and when work related injury or illness occurs, to treat these conditions. This field combines preventive and therapeutic health services and, as the numbers of persons in many occupations are known fairly precisely, it provides good opportunities for epidemiologic studies.[1] Bernadino Ramazzini (1633–1714) is regarded as the "father of occupation medicine," having published *De Morbis Artificum* (On the Diseases of Workers) in 1700.

[1] Monson RR. *Occupational Epidemiology*, 2nd ed. Boca Raton, FL: CRC Press, 1990.

OCCURRENCE (Syn: frequency) In epidemiology, a general term describing the frequency of a disease or other attribute or event in a population without distinguishing between INCIDENCE and PREVALENCE.

ODDS The ratio of the probability of occurrence of an event to that of nonoccurrence, or the ratio of the probability that something is so to the probability that it is not so. If 60 smokers develop a chronic cough and 40 do not, the odds among these 100 smokers in favor of developing a cough are 60:40, or 1.5; this may be contrasted with the probability that these smokers will develop a cough, which is 60/100 or 0.6.

ODDS RATIO (Syn: cross-product ratio, relative odds) The ratio of two odds. The term *odds* is defined differently according to the situation under discussion. Consider the following notation for the distribution of a binary exposure and a disease in a population or a sample.

	Exposed	Unexposed
Disease	a	b
No disease	c	d

The odds ratio (cross-product ratio) is ad/bc.

The *exposure-odds ratio* for a set of case control data is the ratio of the odds in favor of exposure among the cases (a/b) to the odds in favor of exposure among noncases (c/d). This reduces to ad/bc. With incident cases, unbiased subject selection, and a "rare" disease (say, under 2% cumulative incidence rate over the study period), ad/bc is an approximate estimate of the RISK RATIO. With incident cases, unbiased subject selection, and DENSITY SAMPLING of controls ad/bc is an estimate of the ratio of the person-time incidence rates (FORCE OF MORBIDITY) in the exposed and unexposed (no rarity assumption is required for this).

The *disease-odds (rate-odds) ratio* for a cohort or cross section is the ratio of the odds in favor of disease among the exposed (a/c) to the odds in favor of disease among the unexposed b/d). This reduces to ad/bc and hence is equal to the exposure-odds ratio for the cohort or cross section.

The *prevalence-odds ratio* refers to an odds ratio derived cross-sectionally, as, for example, an odds ratio derived from studies of prevalent (rather than incident) cases.

The *risk-odds ratio* is the ratio of the odds in favor of getting disease, if exposed, to the odds in favor of getting disease if not exposed. The odds ratio derived from a cohort study is an estimate of this. See also CASE CONTROL STUDY.

ONCOGENE A gene that can cause neoplastic transformation of a cell; oncogenes are slightly transformed equivalents of normal genes.

OPEN-ENDED QUESTION A question that allows respondents to answer in their own words rather than according to a predetermined set of possible responses—i.e., a closed-end question. Open-ended questions can be difficult to code and classify for statistical analysis.

ONE-TAIL TEST A statistical significance test based on the assumption that the data have only one possible direction of variability.

OPERATIONAL DEFINITION A definition embodying criteria that are used to identify and classify individual members of a set.

OPERATIONAL RESEARCH The systematic study, by observation and experiment, of the working of a system, e.g., health services, with a view to improvement.

OPERATIONS RESEARCH
1. The fitting of models to data, or the designing of models.
2. Synonym for OPERATIONAL RESEARCH.

OPPORTUNISTIC INFECTION Infection with organism(s) that are normally innocuous, e.g., commensals in the human, but become pathogenic when the body's immunologic defenses are compromised, as happens in the acquired immunodeficiency syndrome (AIDS).

ORDINAL SCALE See MEASUREMENT SCALE.

ORDINATE The distance of a point, *P,* from the horizontal or *x* axis of a graph, measured along the vertical or *y* axis. See also ABSCISSA; GRAPH.

OUTCOMES All the possible results that may stem from exposure to a causal factor, or from preventive or therapeutic interventions; all identified changes in health status arising as a consequence of the handling of a health problem. See also CAUSALITY; CAUSATION OF DISEASE, FACTORS IN.

OUTLIERS Observations differing so widely from the rest of the data as to lead one to suspect that a gross error may have been committed, or suggesting that these values come from a different population.

OUTBREAK An epidemic limited to localized increase in the incidence of a disease, e.g., in a village, town, or closed institution; *upsurge* is sometimes used as a euphemism for outbreak.

OUTCOME RESEARCH Research on outcomes of interventions. This is a large part of the work of clinical epidemiologists.

OUTPUT The immediate result of professional or institutional health care activities, usually expressed as units of service, e.g., patient hospital days, outpatient visits, laboratory tests performed.

OVERADJUSTMENT Selection of statistical criteria for adjustment uninformed by clinical or common sense. It can obscure a true effect or create an apparent effect when none exists.[1]

[1] Breslow N. Design and analysis of case-control studies. *Annu Rev Public Health* 1982; 3:29–54.

OVERCROWDING This sociodemographic term is variously defined. The UK Office of Population Censuses and Surveys (OPCS) uses an *index of overcrowding,* defined as the number of persons in private households living at a density greater than one person per room, as a proportion of all persons in private households.

OVERMATCHING A situation that may arise when groups are matched. Several varieties can be distinguished:
1. The matching procedure partially or completely obscures evidence of a true causal association between the independent and dependent variables. Overmatching may occur if the matching variable is involved in, or is closely connected with, the mechanism whereby the independent variable affects the de-

pendent variable. The matching variable may be an intermediate cause in the causal chain or it may be strongly affected by, or a consequence of, such an intermediate cause.

2. The matching procedure uses one or more unnecessary matching variables, e.g., variables that have no causal effect or influence on the dependent variable, and hence cannot confound the relationship between the independent and dependent variables.

3. The matching process is unduly elaborate, involving the use of numerous matching variables and/or insisting on very close similarity with respect to specific matching variables. This leads to difficulty in finding suitable controls. See also MATCHING.

OVERVIEW See METAANALYSIS.

OVERWINTERING See VECTOR-BORNE INFECTION.

P

P, (PROBABILITY) VALUE The probability that a test statistic would be as extreme as or more extreme than observed if the null hypothesis were true. The letter P, followed by the abbreviation n.s. (not significant) or by the symbol < (less than) and a decimal notation such as 0.01, 0.05, is a statement of the probability that the difference observed could have occurred by chance if the groups were really alike, i.e., under the NULL HYPOTHESIS.

Investigators may arbitrarily set their own significance levels, but in most biomedical and epidemiologic work, a study result whose probability value is less than 5% ($P < 0.05$) or 1% ($P < 0.01$) is considered sufficiently unlikely to have occurred by chance to justify the designation "statistically significant." See also STATISTICAL SIGNIFICANCE.

PAIRED SAMPLES In a CLINICAL TRIAL, pairs of subject patients may be studied. One member of each pair receives the experimental regimen, and the other receives a suitably designated control regimen. Pairing should be based on a prognostic variable such as age.

Pairing may similarly be used in a CASE CONTROL STUDY or in a COHORT STUDY. See also MATCHING.

PANDEMIC An epidemic occurring over a very wide area, crossing international boundaries and usually affecting a large number of people.

PANEL STUDY A combination of cross-sectional and cohort methods, in which the investigator conducts a series of cross-sectional studies of the same individuals or study sample. This method of study permits changes in one variable to be related to changes in other variables. See also NESTED CASE CONTROL STUDY.

PARADIGM A typical example, a pattern of thought or conceptualization, an overall way of regarding phenomena within which scientists normally work. A paradigm may dictate what form of explanation will be found acceptable, but a science may change paradigms.[1] In many contexts in which it is used, the term is ambiguous and vague.

[1] Kuhn T. *The Structure of Scientific Revolutions.* Chicago: University of Chicago Press, 1962.

PARAMETER In mathematics, a constant in a formula or model; in statistics and epidemiology, a measureable characteristic of a population.

PARAMETRIC TEST A statistical test that depends upon assumption(s) about the distribution of the data, e.g., that these are normally distributed.

PARASITE An animal or vegetable organism that lives on or in another and derives its nourishment therefrom. An obligate parasite is one that cannot lead an independent nonparasitic existence. A facultative parasite is one that is capable of either parasitic or independent existence.

PARASITE COUNT See WORM COUNT.

PARASITE DENSITY The collective degree of parasitemia in a population, calculated by the use of either the geometric mean or the weighted average of the individual parasite counts; e.g., by using a frequency distribution based on a geometric progression.

PARATENIC HOST (Syn: transport host) A second, third, or subsequent intermediate host of a parasite, in which the parasite does not undergo any development or replication but remains, usually encysted, until the paratenic host is ingested by the definitive host of the parasite.

PARITY The status of a woman as regards the fact of having borne viable children. The number of full-term children previously borne by a woman, excluding miscarriages or abortions in early pregnancy but including stillbirths.

PARTICIPANT OBSERVATION A method used in the social sciences in which the research worker (observer) is a member of the group being studied. Epidemiologists distrust the method on the grounds that objectivity of the observations may be compromised.

PARTICULARIZATION A method of analysis opposite to generalization or abstraction. It focuses on the specificity of a number of facts and illustrates an issue through the use of example.

PASSAGE The transfer of microorganisms from human to animal host(s) either directly or via laboratory culture; in the laboratory, this procedure is used to establish the Henle–Koch postulates.

PASSENGER VARIABLE A variable that varies systematically with the dependent variable under study without being causally related to it. A third (explanatory) variable, the common cause of both the dependent and the passenger variable, "explains" or accounts for their association.

PASSIVE SMOKING See INVOLUNTARY SMOKING, ENVIRONMENTAL TOBACCO SMOKE.

PASTEURIZATION The process of heat-treating milk or other perishable foodstuffs to kill pathogens. Developed by and named for the great French bacteriologist Louis Pasteur (1822–1895).

PATH ANALYSIS A mode of analysis involving assumptions about the direction of causal relationships between linked sequences and configurations of variables. This permits the analyst to construct and test the appropriateness of alternative models (in the form of a path diagram) of the causal relations that may exist within the array of variables included in the finite system studied. Identification of the less probable sequences of causal pathways may permit them to be eliminated from further consideration.

PATHOGEN Organism capable of causing disease (literally, causing a pathological process).

PATHOGENESIS The postulated mechanisms by which the etiologic agent produces disease. The difference between ETIOLOGY and pathogenesis should be noted: The etiology of a disease or disability consists of the postulated causes that initiate the pathogenetic mechanisms; control of these causes might lead to prevention of the disease.

PATHOGENICITY The property of an organism that determines the extent to which overt disease is produced in an infected population, or the power of an organism to produce disease. Also used to describe comparable properties of toxic chemicals, etc. Pathogenicity of infectious agents is measured by the ratio of the number of persons developing clinical illness to the number exposed to infection. See also VIRULENCE, with which pathogenicity is sometimes confused.

PEARSON'S PRODUCT MOMENT CORRELATION See CORRELATION COEFFICIENT.

PEDIGREE A diagram showing the ancestral relationships and transmission of genetic traits over several generations of a family.

PEER REVIEW Process of review of research proposals, manuscripts submitted for publication, abstracts submitted for presentation at scientific meetings, whereby these are judged for scientific and technical merit by other scientists in the same field. The term also refers to review of clinical performance, when it is a form of medical AUDIT.

PENETRANCE The frequency, expressed as a percentage, with which individuals of a given phenotype manifest at least some degree of a specific mutant phenotype associated with a trait. See also GENETIC PENETRANCE.

PERCEIVED NEED A felt need. The term usually refers to need for health care that is felt by the person or community concerned but which may not be perceived by health professionals.

PERCENTILE The set of divisions that produce exactly 100 equal parts in a series of continuous values, such as children's heights or weights. Thus a child above the 90th percentile has a greater value for height or weight than over 90% of all in the series.

PERINATAL MORTALITY Literally, mortality around the time of birth. Conventionally this time is limited to the period between 28 weeks gestation and one week postnatal. However, as the following discussion indicates, other factors, especially the weight of the fetus, should be considered. The *Ninth (1975) Revision of the International Classification of Diseases* includes the following:

Perinatal mortality statistics
It is recommended that national perinatal statistics should include all fetuses and infants delivered weighing at least 500 g (or, when birth weight is unavailable, the corresponding gestational age [22 weeks] or body length [25 cm crown—heel]), whether alive or dead. It is recognized that legal requirements in many countries may set different criteria for registration purposes, but it is hoped that countries will arrange the registration or reporting procedures in such a way that the events required for inclusion in the statistics can be identified easily. It is further recommended that less mature fetuses and infants should be excluded from perinatal statistics unless there are legal or other valid reasons to the contrary.

It is recommended above that national statistics would include fetuses and infants weighing between 500 g and 1000 g both for their inherent value and because their inclusion improves the completeness of reporting at 1000 g and over.

Inclusion of this group of very immature births, however, disrupts international comparisons because of differences in national practices concerning their registration. Another factor affecting international comparisons is that all live-born infants, irrespective of birth weight, are included in the calculation of rates, whereas some lower limit of maturity is applied to infants born dead.

In order to eliminate these factors, it is recommended that countries should present, solely for international comparisons, "standard perinatal statistics" in which both the numerator and denominator of all rates are restricted to fetuses and infants weighing 1000 g or more (or, where birth weight is unavailable, the corresponding gestational age [28 weeks] or body length [25 cm crown-heel]).

The Conference for the tenth revision (ICD-10) made no changes to these definitions.

PERINATAL MORTALITY RATE In most industrially developed nations, this is defined as

$$\text{Perinatal mortality rate} = \frac{\text{Fetal deaths (28 weeks + of gestation) + postnatal deaths (first week)}}{\text{Fetal deaths (28 weeks + of gestation) + live births)}} \times 1000$$

The WHO's definition, more appropriate in nations with less well established vital records, is

$$\text{Perinatal mortality rate} = \frac{\text{Late fetal deaths (28 weeks + of gestation) + postnatal deaths (first week)}}{\text{Live births in a year}} \times 1000$$

Note the differences in denominator of the perinatal mortality rate as defined by the WHO and in industrially developed nations. This makes international comparison difficult. The WHO Expert Committee on the Prevention of Perinatal Mortality and Morbidity (1970) recommended a more precise formulation: "Late fetal and early neonatal deaths weighing over 1000 g at birth expressed as a ratio per 1000 live births weighing over 1000 g at birth."

PERIODIC (MEDICAL) EXAMINATIONS Assessment of health status conducted at predetermined intervals, e.g., annually or at specified milestones in life such as infancy, school entry, preemployment, or preretirement. This form of medical examination generally follows a formal protocol, e.g., employing a set of structured questions and/or a predetermined set of laboratory tests.

PERIOD OF COMMUNICABILITY See COMMUNICABLE PERIOD.

PERMISSIBLE EXPOSURE LIMIT (PEL) An occupational health standard to safeguard workers against dangerous substances in the workplace. See SAFETY STANDARDS.

PERSONAL HEALTH CARE Those services to individuals that are performed on a one-to-one basis by a health care worker for the purpose of maintaining or restoring health.

PERSONAL MONITORING DEVICE An instrument attached to a person to measure the exposure of that person to hazardous substance(s).

PERSON-TIME A measurement combining persons and time, used as denominator in person-time incidence and mortality rates. It is the sum of individual units of time that the persons in the study population have been exposed to the condition of interest. A variant is person-distance, e.g., as in passenger-kilometers. The most frequently used person-time is person-years. With this approach, each subject contributes only as many years of observation to the population at risk as he is actually observed; if he leaves after 1 year, he contributes 1 person-year; if after 10, 10 person-years. The method can be used to measure incidence over extended and variable time periods.

PERSON-TIME INCIDENCE RATE (Syn: interval incidence density) A measure of the incidence rate of an event, e.g., a disease or death, in a population at risk, given by

$$\frac{\text{Number of events occurring during the interval}}{\text{Number of person-time units at risk observed during the interval}}$$

PERSON-TO-PERSON SPREAD OF DISEASE See TRANSMISSION OF INFECTION.

PERSON-YEARS See PERSON-TIME.

PHARMACOEPIDEMIOLOGY The study of the distribution and determinants of drug-related events in populations and the application of this study to efficaceous drug treatment.

PHYSICIAN (Syn: medical practitioner, doctor) Professional person qualified by education and authorized by law to practice medicine.

PIE CHART A circular diagram divided into segments, each representing a category or subset of data. The amount for each category is proportional to the angle subtended at the center of the circle and hence to the area of the sector.

When several pie charts are used to describe several populations, the area of each circle is proportional to the size of the population it represents.

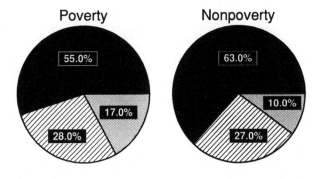

Adequately vaccinated: 3+ doses inactivated poliovirus vaccine (IPV) and/or 3 doses oral poliovirus vaccine (OPV).

Inadequately vaccinated: Some poliovirus vaccine, but < 3 doses of IPV and/or < 3 doses of OPV.

Not vaccinated: No vaccine given.

Pie chart. Proportions adequately vaccinated against poliovirus by financial status. From Teutsch and Churchill, op. cit. With permission.

PILOT INVESTIGATION, STUDY A small-scale test of the methods and procedures to be used on a larger scale if the pilot study demonstrates that these methods and procedures can work.

PLACEBO, PLACEBO EFFECT An inert medication or procedure. The placebo effect (usually but not necessarily beneficial) is attributable to the expectation that the regimen will have an effect, i.e., the effect is due to the power of suggestion. See also HALO EFFECT.

POINT SOURCE EPIDEMIC See EPIDEMIC, COMMON SOURCE.

POISSON DISTRIBUTION A distribution function used to describe the occurrence of rare events or to describe the sampling distribution of isolated counts in a continuum of time or space (e.g., sample counts of radioactive disintegration per minute). The number of events has a Poisson distribution with parameter λ (lambda) if the probability of observing k events ($k = 0, 1, \ldots$) is equal to

$$p(x = k) = \frac{e^{-\lambda}\lambda^k}{k!}$$

where e is the base of natural logarithm, 2.7183. . . . The mean and variance of the distribution are both equal to λ. This distribution is used in modeling person-time incidence rates.

POLLUTANT Any undesirable solid, liquid, or gaseous matter in a solid, liquid, or gaseous environmental medium.

POLLUTION Any undesirable modification of air, water, or food by substance(s) that are toxic or may have adverse effects on health or that are offensive though not necessarily harmful to health.

POLYGENIC INHERITANCE The transmission of a phenotypic trait whose expression depends upon the additive effect of a number of genes.

PONDERAL INDEX The anthropometric index of body mass. Defined as height divided by the cube root of the body weight. The BODY MASS INDEX is generally regarded as a better index of body mass.

POPULATION

1. All the inhabitants of a given country or area considered together; the number of inhabitants of a given country or area.
2. (In sampling) The whole collection of units (the "UNIVERSE") from which a sample may be drawn; not necessarily a population of persons; the units may be institutions, records, or events. The sample is intended to give results that are representative of the whole population.

POPULATION ATTRIBUTABLE RISK (PAR) This term is used by many epidemiologists[1-3] in preference to the terms ATTRIBUTABLE FRACTION (POPULATION) or ETIOLOGIC FRACTION (POPULATION). It is the incidence of a disease in a population that is associated with (attributable to) exposure to the risk factor. It is often expressed as a percentage. It is calculated by similar methods to those described for attributable fraction (population), i.e.,

$$PAR\% = \frac{P_e(I_e - I_u)}{P_t \times I_t} \times 100$$

where

P_e = number of persons exposed
P_t = persons in the population
I_e = incidence rate among the exposed
I_u = incidence rate among the unexposed
I_t = incidence rate for the total population

In a case control study, PAR can be estimated in various ways; Cole and Mac-Mahon[3] gave the following formula:

$$PAR\% = \frac{P_e(RR - 1)}{1 + P_e(RR - 1)} \times 100$$

where

P_e = proportion of controls exposed
RR = relative risk for exposed, compared to risk of 1 for the unexposed.

[1] MacMahon B, Pugh TF. *Epidemiology; Principles and Methods.* Boston: Little, Brown, 1970.
[2] Fletcher RH, Fletcher SW, Wagner EH. *Clinical Epidemiology—the Essentials.* Baltimore: Williams & Wilkins, 1982.
[3] Cole P, MacMahon B. Attributable risk percent in case-control studies. *Br J Prev Soc Med* 1971; 25:242–244.

POPULATION ATTRIBUTABLE RISK PERCENT This is the attributable fraction in the population, expressed as a percentage. See also ATTRIBUTABLE FRACTION (POPULATION).

POPULATION BASED Pertaining to a general population defined by geopolitical boundaries; this population is the denominator and/or the sampling frame.

POPULATION DYNAMICS Changes in the structure of a population; loosely used as a synonym for DEMOGRAPHY.

POPULATION EXCESS RATE A measure of the amount of disease associated with exposure to a putative cause of the disease in the population. It is the difference between the rates of disease in the entire population and among the nonexposed.

POPULATION GENETICS Study of the genetic composition of populations. The main aim is to estimate gene frequencies and detect selective factors in the environment that influence these frequencies.

POPULATION MEDICINE See COMMUNITY MEDICINE.

POPULATION MOMENTUM In a growing population, the phenomenon of continuing population growth beyond the time when replacement-level fertility has been achieved, because of the increasing size of childbearing and younger age cohorts, resulting from higher fertility and/or falling mortality in preceding years.

POPULATION PYRAMID A graphic presentation of the age and sex composition of the population. The population pyramid is constructed by computing the percentage

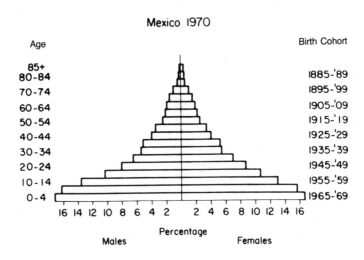

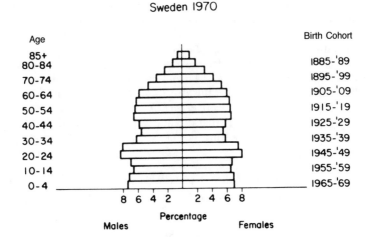

Population pyramids.
Top: High fertility, low proportion survive to old age (Mexico).
Bottom: Low fertility, high proportion survive to old age (Sweden).
From Last JM (Ed): *Maxcy-Rosenau Public Health and Preventive Medicine,*
11th ed. New York: Appleton-Century-Crofts, 1986.

distribution of a population, simultaneously cross-classified by sex and age. The percentage that each female age group is of the total is plotted on the right and the corresponding percentages for males are plotted on the left. Sometimes the pyramid is constructed using absolute numbers in each age and sex group, rather than proportions. A population pyramid is intended to provide a quick overall comprehension of age and sex structure in the population. A population whose pyramid has a broad base and narrow apex may be identified as a high-fertility population. Changing shape over time reflects the changing composition of the population, associated with changes in fertility and mortality at each age.

Since the figure is two dimensional, the word *pyramid* is incorrectly used, but the more accurate word *profile* has never caught on.

POPULATION, STUDY The group selected for investigation.

POPULATION, TARGET The group from which a study population is selected.

POSTERIOR ODDS, POSTERIOR PROBABILITY Probability calculated after reference to results of a study. See BAYES' THEOREM.

POSTMARKETING SURVEILLANCE A procedure implemented after a drug has been licensed for public use, designed to provide information on the actual use of the drug for a given indication, and on the occurrence of side effects, adverse reactions, etc. A method for epidemiologic study of adverse drug reactions.

POSTNEONATAL MORTALITY RATE The number of infant deaths between 28 days and 1 year of age in a given year per 1000 live births in that year. It is an important rate to monitor in developing countries where older infants frequently die of infections and malnutrition.

POTENCY The strength of a particular drug, toxin, or hazard; the ratio of the dose of a standard amount required to elicit a specific response, to the dose of the test agent that elicits the same response.

POTENTIAL YEARS OF LIFE LOST (PYLL) A measure of the relative impact of various diseases and lethal forces on society. PYLL highlights the loss to society as a result of youthful or early deaths. The figure for potential years of life lost due to a particular cause is the sum, over all persons dying from that cause, of the years that these persons would have lived had they experienced normal life expectation. The concept derives from Petty's *Political Arithmetic* (1687) and is elaborated upon in Dublin and Lotka's *Money Value of a Man* (1930).

POWER The ability of a study to demonstrate an association if one exists. The power of a study is determined by several factors, including the frequency of the condition under study, the magnitude of the effect, the study design, and sample size. Mathematically, power is $1 - \beta$ (type II error). A characteristic of a statistical hypothesis test, denoting the probability that the null hypothesis will be rejected if it is indeed false. See also ERROR. Resolving power is the comparable property of individual measurements.

PRAGMATIC STUDY A study whose aim is to improve health status or health care of a specified population, provide a basis for decisions about health care, or evaluate previous actions. See also EXPLANATORY STUDY; COMMUNITY DIAGNOSIS; PROGRAM REVIEW.

PRECISION

1. The quality of being sharply defined or stated. One measure of precision is the number of distinguishable alternatives from which a measurement was selected, sometimes indicated by the number of significant digits in the measurement. Another measure of precision is the standard error of measurement, the standard deviation of a series of replicate determinations of the

same quantity. Precision does not imply accuracy. See also MEASUREMENT, TERMINOLOGY OF.

2. In statistics, precision is defined as the inverse of the variance of a measurement or estimate.

PRECURSOR A condition or state preceding pathological onset of a disease; sometimes detectable by SCREENING; may be identified as a RISK MARKER.

PREDICTIVE VALUE In screening and diagnostic tests, the probability that a person with a positive test is a true positive (i.e., does have the disease) is referred to as the "predictive value of a positive test." The predictive value of a negative test is the probability that a person with a negative test does not have the disease. The predictive value of a screening test is determined by the sensitivity and specificity of the test, and by the prevalence of the condition for which the test is used. See also SCREENING; SENSITIVITY AND SPECIFICITY.

PREGNANCY-RELATED DEATH See MATERNAL MORTALITY

PREMUNITION A term used mainly in the epidemiology of parastic diseases, especially malaria. It signifies a state of resistance, in a host harboring a parasite, to superinfection by a parasite of the same species. This state is dependent on the continued survival of parasites in the body and disappears after their elimination. It may be complete or partial.

PREPATENT PERIOD In parasitology, the period equivalent to the incubation period of microbial infections; the corresponding phase may be biologically different from microbial multiplication when the invading organism is a multicellular parasite that undergoes developmental stages in the host.

PRESCRIPTIVE SCREENING See SCREENING.

PREVALENCE The number of events, e.g., instances of a given disease or other condition, in a given population at a designated time; sometimes used to mean PREVALENCE RATE. When used without qualification, the term usually refers to the situation at a specified point in time (point prevalence). Note that this is a number, not a rate.

Prevalence, annual The total number of persons with the disease or attribute at any time during a year. An occasionally used index. It includes cases of the disease arising before but extending into or through the year as well as those having their inception during the year.

Prevalence, lifetime The total number of persons known to have had the disease or attribute for at least part of their lives.

Prevalence, period The total number of persons known to have had the disease or attribute at any time during a specified period.

Prevalence, point The number of persons with a disease or an attribute at a specified point in time.

PREVALENCE "RATE" (RATIO) The total number of all individuals who have an attribute or disease at a particular time (or during a particular period) divided by the population at risk of having the attribute or disease at this point in time or midway through the period. A problem may arise with calculating period prevalence rates because of the difficulty of defining the most appropriate denominator. This is a proportion, not a rate. See also PREVALENCE.

PREVALENCE STUDY See CROSS-SECTIONAL STUDY.

PREVENTABLE FRACTION (population) In a situation in which exposure to a given factor is believed to protect against a disease (or other outcome), the preventable fraction in the population is the proportion of the disease (in the population) that would be prevented if the whole population were exposed to the factor. This value must be interpreted with caution, as part or all of the apparent protective effect may be due to other factors associated with the apparent protective factor.

In a study of a total population, the preventable fraction (population) is computed as

$$(I_p - I_e)/I_p,$$

where I_p is the incidence rate of the disease (or other outcome) in the population and I_e is the incidence rate in the exposed persons in the population.

PREVENTED FRACTION (population) In a situation in which exposure to a given factor is believed to protect against a disease (or other outcome), the prevented fraction is the proportion of the hypothetical total load of disease (in the population) that has been prevented by exposure to the factor. This value must be interpreted with caution, as part or all of the apparent protective effect may be due to other factors associated with the apparent protective factor.

In a study of a total population, the prevented fraction is computed as

$$(I_u - I_p)/I_u,$$

where I_p is the rate of the disease in the population and I_u is the rate among people unexposed to the factor.

PREVENTION The goals of medicine are to promote health, to preserve health, to restore health when it is impaired, and to minimize suffering and distress. These goals are embodied in the word *prevention,* which is easiest to define in the context of levels, customarily called primary, secondary, and tertiary prevention. Authorities on PREVENTIVE MEDICINE do not agree on the precise boundaries between these levels, nor on how many levels can be distinguished, but the differences of opinion are semantic rather than substantive.

An epidemiologic interpretation of the distinction between primary and secondary prevention is that primary prevention is aimed at reducing incidence of disease and other departures from good health, secondary prevention aims to reduce prevalence by shortening the duration, and tertiary prevention is aimed at reducing the number or the impact of complications.

Primary prevention can be defined as the protection of health by personal and communitywide effects, e.g., preserving good nutritional status, physical fitness, and emotional well-being, immunizing against infectious diseases, and making the environment safe. (But see also HEALTH PROMOTION.)

Secondary prevention can be defined as the measures available to individuals and populations for the early detection and prompt and effective intervention to correct departures from good health.

Tertiary prevention consists of the measures available to reduce or eliminate long-term impairments and disabilities, minimize suffering caused by existing departures from good health, and to promote the patient's adjustment to irremediable conditions. This extends the concept of prevention into the field of rehabilitation.

PREVENTION PARADOX A preventive measure that brings large benefits to the community but may offer little to most participating persons.[1] For example, to prevent one death due to a motor vehicle accident, many hundreds of people must wear seat belts. Similarly, to reduce the death rate from lung cancer, many people must refrain from or cease smoking; but only some who have been exposed to tobacco smoke will die prematurely of smoking-related diseases.

[1] Rose GA: *The Strategy of Preventive Medicine.* Oxford, England: Oxford Medical Publications 1992.

PREVENTIVE MEDICINE The application of preventive measures by clinical practitioners. A specialized field of medical practice composed of distinct disciplines that utilize skills focusing on the health of defined populations in order to promote and maintain health and well-being and prevent disease, disability, and premature death.

In addition to the knowledge of basic and clinical sciences and the skills common to all physicians, the distinctive aspects of preventive medicine include knowledge of and competence in biostatistics; epidemiology; administration, including planning, organization, management, financing, and evaluation of health programs; environmental health; application of social and behavioral factors in health and disease; and the application of primary, secondary, and tertiary prevention measures within clinical medicine. (The above is the definition and description of the field that has been adopted by the American College of Preventive Medicine; other items ought to be added, i.e., health promotion, health education, and nutrition).

PRIMARY CASE The individual who introduces the disease into the family or group under study. Not necessarily the first diagnosed case in a family or group. See also INDEX CASE.

PRIMARY HEALTH CARE

1. Health care that begins at the time of first encounter between a patient and a provider of health care; An alternative term is *primary medical care*.[1]
2. The WHO definition of primary health care includes much more: Primary health care is essential health care made accessible at a cost the country and the community can afford, with methods that are practical, scientifically sound, and socially acceptable. Everyone in the community should have access to it, and everyone should be involved in it. Related sectors should also be involved in it in addition to the health sector. At the very least it should include education of the community on the health problems prevalent and on methods of preventing health problems from arising or of controlling them; the promotion of adequate supplies of food and of proper nutrition; sufficient safe water and basic sanitation; maternal and child health care including family planning; the prevention and control of locally endemic diseases; immunization against the main infectious diseases; appropriate treatment of common diseases and injuries; and the provision of essential drugs.[2]

[1] Starfield B. *Primary Care: Concept, Evaluation and Policy.* New York: Oxford University Press, 1992.
[2] *Glossary of Terms Used in the Health for All Series No. 1–8.* Geneva: WHO, 1984.

PRIMORDIAL PREVENTION This term is advocated by some authors to describe elimination of risk factors, precursors, genetic counseling to avoid genetically determined conditions, etc., in contrast to primary prevention by reducing risks of exposure.

PRINCIPAL COMPONENT ANALYSIS A statistical method to simplify the description of a set of interrelated variables. Its general objectives are data reduction and interpretation; there is no separation into dependent and independent variables; the original set of correlated variables is transformed into a smaller set of uncorrelated variables called the principal components. Often used as the first step in a factor analysis.

PRION Viruslike particle, an infectious protein, to which several so-called slow virus diseases—including kuru, Creutzfeldt-Jakob disease, scrapie, and bovine spongiform encephalopathy—are attributed. The word was coined in 1982 by S. Prusiner, from *pro*teinaceous *in*fectious particles, reversing the order of the vowels. See also SLOW VIRUS.

PRIOR PROBABILITY Probability calculated or estimated from theory or belief, before a study is done. See BAYES' THEOREM.

PRIVACY The state of being undisturbed or free from public attention. Privacy and CONFIDENTIALITY are protected by public interest groups and in some nations by privacy commissioners; the safeguards can affect epidemiologic research requiring access to personal, private information. The rules, regulations, and laws governing privacy and access to health-related information vary and change frequently; constant dialogue among the parties concerned is required.

PROBABILITY

1. The limit of the relative frequency of an event in a sequence of N random trials as N approaches infinity, i.e., the limit of

$$\frac{\text{Number of occurrence of the event}}{N}$$

2. A measure, ranging from zero to 1, of the degree of belief in a hypothesis or statement.

PROBABILITY DENSITY The frequency distribution of a continuous random variable.

PROBABILITY DISTRIBUTION For a discrete random variable, the function that gives the probabilities that the variable equals each of a sequence of possible values. Examples include the binomial and Poisson distributions. For a continuous random variable, often used synonymously with the probability density function.

PROBABILITY SAMPLE (Syn: random sample) See SAMPLE.

PROBABILITY THEORY The branch of mathematics dealing with the purely logical properties of probability. Its theorems underlie most statistical methods.

PROBAND See PROPOSITUS.

PROBLEM-ORIENTED MEDICAL RECORD (POMR) A medical record in which the patient's history, physical findings, laboratory results, etc., are organized to give a cumulative record of problems, e.g., hemoptysis, rather than disease, e.g., pneumonia. The record includes subjective, objective, and significant negative information, discussions and conclusions, and diagnostic and treatment plans with respect to each problem. The record, which was developed by Lawrence Weed,[1] contrasts with the traditional medical record, which is less formally organized, usually recording all information from each source (history, physical, and laboratory findings) together without regard to the problems the information describes.

Since the problems may not be described in terms of conventional disease labels, their classification and counting for epidemiologic purposes are sometimes difficult. The INTERNATIONAL CLASSIFICATION OF HEALTH PROBLEMS IN PRIMARY CARE (ICHPPC) is an attempt to overcome this difficulty.

[1] Weed LL. Medical records that guide and teach. *N Engl J Med* 1968; 278:593–600, 652–657.

PROCATARCTIC CAUSE A term used by epidemiologists of the late 19th and early 20th centuries, to describe predisposing causes associated with habits of life.

PRODUCT LIMIT METHOD See KAPLAN–MEIER ESTIMATE.

PROFESSIONAL ACTIVITY STUDY (PAS) The HOSPITAL DISCHARGE ABSTRACT SYSTEM, which covers many acute short-stay hospitals in the United States. It provides regularly published statistical tables arranged according to hospital service, diagnostic category, etc., giving details on diagnostic and therapeutic procedures, length of stay, and outcome.

PROFILE PLOT (Syn: barycentric coordinates) A graphical method of data presentation used when several categories add to 100%; it permits the categories to be plotted on a plane surface using coordinates running inward at right angles from each side of an equilateral polyhedron.

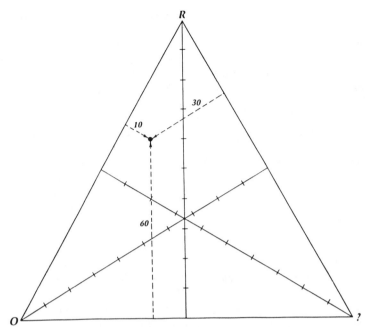

Profile plot. Reprinted by permission of The Massachusetts Medical Society, from Bailar, J. C., Mosteller, F., eds., *Medical Uses of Statistics,* Boston, NEJM Books, 1986. Figure 1, p. 275. Copyright 1986. Massachusetts Medical Society.

PROGRAM
1. A (formal) set of procedures to conduct an activity, e.g., control of malaria.
2. An ordered list of instructions directing a computer to carry out a desired sequence of operations. The objective is normally the solution of a problem.

PROGRAM EVALUATION AND REVIEW TECHNIQUES (PERT) A work-scheduling method that uses ALGORITHMS and also enunciates general principles of procedure for allocating resources. Calls for listing specific tasks to be completed and the resources—personnel, equipment, supplies, and other items—that will be needed, along with their costs, a time chart indicating when each component task is to begin and end, giving interim accomplishment levels during that period, and a specification of times for interim review of the progress of the plan.

PROGRAM REVIEW An evaluative study of a specific health program operating in a specific setting, performed to provide a basis for decisions concerning the operation of the program.

PROGRAM TRIAL An experimental or quasi-experimental evaluative study of a (health) program.

PROLECTIVE Pertaining to data collected by planning in advance. Contrast *retrolective.* The terms *prolective* and *retrolective,* coined by AR Feinstein,[1] are said to describe more precisely the actions of research workers than the common terms *prospective* and *retrospective.*

[1] *Clin Pharmacol Ther* 1981; 30:564–577.

PROPORTION A type of ratio in which the numerator is included in the denominator. The ratio of a part to the whole, expressed as a "decimal fraction" (e.g., 0.2), as a "vulgar fraction" (1/5), or as a percentage (20%). By definition, a proportion (*p*) must be in the range (decimal) $0.0 \leqslant p \leqslant 1.0$. Since numerator and denominator have the same dimension, any dimensional contents cancel out, and a proportion is a dimensionless quantity. Where numerator and denominator are based upon counts rather than upon measurements, the originals are also dimensionless, although it should be understood that proportions can be used for measured quantities, e.g., the skin area of the lower limb is x percent of the total skin area, as well as for counts, e.g., 15% of the population died. A prevalence rate is a count-based proportion. The nondimensionality of a proportion, and its range limitations, do not necessarily apply to other kinds of ratios, of which "proportion" is a subset. See also RATE; RATIO.

PROPORTIONAL HAZARDS MODEL (Syn: Cox model) a statistical MODEL in SURVIVAL ANALYSIS developed by D. R. Cox in 1972 asserting that the effect of the study factors on the HAZARD RATE in the study population is multiplicative and does not change over time. For example, the model for two factors x_1 and x_2 asserts that the rate at time t λ (t), is given by

$$e^{\beta_1 x_1 + \beta_2 x_2} \lambda_0(t)$$

where $\lambda_0(t)$ is the rate when $x_1 = x_2 = 0$, and e is the (natural) exponential function.

PROPORTIONAL MORTALITY RATIO The proportion of observed deaths from a specified condition in a defined population, divided by the proportion of deaths expected from this condition in a standard population, expressed either on an age-specific basis or after age adjustment. Unlike the STANDARDIZED MORTALITY RATIO, it does not require data on the age composition of the population but only on the deaths. The acronym, PMR, is preferably avoided because the same initial letters can stand for perinatal mortality rate.

PROPOSITUS (Syn: proband) The family member who first draws attention to a (genetic) pedigree of a given trait. The INDEX CASE in a genetic study.

PROSPECTIVE STUDY See COHORT STUDY.

PROTOCOL The plan, or set of steps, to be followed in a study or investigation or in an intervention program. See also ALGORITHM, CLINICAL.

PROXIMATE DETERMINANT OF FERTILITY Factor having a direct influence on fertility; such factors include age at marriage, breastfeeding, abortion, and contraceptive use.

PUBLICATION BIAS Tendency of editors (and authors) to publish articles containing positive findings, especially "new" results, in contrast to reports that do not yield "significant" results, i.e. results that accord with previously published findings. Publication bias can distort the general belief—e.g., about associations, efficacy of regimens. It can be a particularly important source of bias in METAANALYSIS.[1]

[1] Petitti DB: *Meta-Analysis, Decision Analysis and Cost-Effectiveness Analysis: Methods for Quantitative Synthesis in Medicine.* New York: Oxford University Press, 1994

PUBLIC HEALTH Public health is one of the efforts organized by society to protect, promote, and restore the people's health. It is the combination of sciences, skills, and beliefs that is directed to the maintenance and improvement of the health of all the people through collective or social actions. The programs, services, and institutions involved emphasize the prevention of disease and the health needs of the population as a whole. Public health activities change with changing technology and social values, but the goals remain the same: to reduce the amount of disease, premature death, and disease-produced discomfort and disability in the population. Public health is thus a social institution, a discipline, and a practice.[1] The Acheson Report[2] offered a more succinct definition: The science and art of preventing disease, prolonging life, and promoting health through organized efforts of society.

[1] *Higher Education for Public Health: A Report of the Milbank Memorial Fund Commission.* New York: 1976

[2] *Public Health in England; The Report of the Committee of Inquiry into the Future Development of the Public Health Function.* Cmnd 289. London: HMSO, 1988.

PUBLIC HEALTH MEDICINE The practice of public health by physicians. See SOCIAL MEDICINE.

PUNCH CARD A card on which data are stored by means of holes punched in specified positions; useful in storing, processing, and analyzing data. Edge-punch cards have marginal holes converted to slots by punching so that they can be manually sorted. The commonly used variety of punch cards have 80 columns and 12 rows. In each column of the card there are 12 positions at which holes may be punched, according to a predetermined code. The position of the hole is the means of identifying the value of a variable. Punch cards of this type are sorted mechanically or electrically to provide a rapid means of processing and analyzing data, sometimes of great complexity. The use of punch cards has increasingly been superceded by direct data entry into a computer. See also DATA PROCESSING.

P **VALUE** See *P* (PROBABILITY).

Q

QUALITATIVE DATA Observations or information characterized by measurement on a categorical scale, i.e., a dichotomous or nominal scale, or, if the categories are ordered, an ordinal scale. Examples are sex, hair color, death or survival, and nationality. See also MEASUREMENT SCALE.

QUALITY-ADJUSTED LIFE EXPECTANCY (QALE) A model for clinical decision making in which estimates of impairment or disability are included in the calculation of life expectancy.

QUALITY-ADJUSTED LIFE YEARS (QALY) An adjustment of life expectancy that reduces the overall life expectancy by amounts which reflect the existence of chronic conditions causing impairment, disability, and/or handicap as assessed from health survey data, hospital discharge data, etc. In practice, numerical weights representing severity of residual disability are established by the judgment of patients and health professionals.

QUALITY ASSURANCE System of procedures, checks, audits, and corrective actions to ensure that all research, testing, monitoring, sampling, analysis, and other technical and reporting activities are of the highest achievable quality. The term is used in health services with the same meaning.

QUALITY CONTROL The supervision and control of all operations involved in a process, usually involving sampling and inspection, in order to detect and correct systematic or excessively random variations in quality.

QUALITY OF CARE A level of performance or accomplishment that characterizes the health care provided. Ultimately, measures of the quality of care always depend upon value judgments, but there are ingredients and determinants of quality that can be measured objectively. These ingredients and determinants have been classified by Donabedian[1] into measures of structure (e.g., manpower, facilities), process (e.g., diagnostic and therapeutic procedures), and outcome (e.g., case fatality rates, disability rates, and levels of patient satisfaction with the service). See also HEALTH SERVICES RESEARCH.

[1] Donabedian A. *A Guide to Medical Care Administration.* Vol 2. New York: American Public Health Association, 1969.

QUALITY OF LIFE The degree to which persons perceive themselves able to function physically, emotionally, socially. Contrast HEALTH STATUS, which is an objective measurement. In a general sense, that which makes life worth living. In a more "quantitative" sense, an estimate of remaining life free of impairment, disability, or handicap, as used in the expression QUALITY-ADJUSTED LIFE YEARS. Somewhere between these is an estimate of the utility of life—for instance, in clinical decision analysis, the utility of life that is impaired by a disabling degree of angina pectoris may be compared with that of a life which may be shorter in duration but free of disabling pain as a result of applying therapeutic procedures. Such trade-offs are part of clinical decision analysis. See also UTILITY.

QUANTAL EFFECT (Syn: All-or-none effect) An effect that can be expressed only in binary form, e.g., as "occurring" or "not occurring." (Source: IUPAC Glossary.)

QUANTILES Divisions of a distribution into equal, ordered subgroups. Deciles are tenths; quartiles, quarters; quintiles, fifths; terciles, thirds; and centiles, hundredths.

QUANTITATIVE DATA Data in numerical quantities such as continuous measurements or counts.

QUARANTINE

Restriction of the activities of well persons or animals who have been exposed to a case of communicable disease during its period of communicability (i.e., contacts) to prevent disease transmission during the incubation period if infection should occur.

a) Absolute or complete quarantine: The limitation of freedom of movement of those exposed to a communicable disease for a period of time not longer than the longest usual incubation period of that disease, in such manner as to prevent effective contact with those not so exposed.

b) Modified quarantine: A selective, partial limitation of freedom of movement of contacts, commonly on the basis of known or presumed differences in susceptibility and related to the danger of disease transmission. It may be designed to meet particular situations. Examples are exclusion of children from school, exemption of immune persons from provisions applicable to susceptible persons, or restriction of military populations to the post or to quarters. It includes: Personal surveillance, the practice of close medical or other supervision of contacts in order to permit prompt recognition of infection or illness but without restricting their movements; and Segregation, the separation of some part of a group of persons or domestic animals from the others for special consideration, control or observation—removal of susceptible children to homes of immune persons, or establishment of a sanitary boundary to protect uninfected from infected portions of a population.[1]

The word *quarantine* comes from the Italian *quaranta,* meaning forty. The clinical distinction between isolation and quarantine is that isolation is the procedure for persons already sick, whereas quarantine is often applied to (apparently) healthy contacts. This has legal and ethical implications if apparently healthy persons must submit to restrictions upon their freedom to move at large in society.

See also ISOLATION.

[1] Benenson AS, ed. *Control of Communicable Disease in Man,* 15th ed. Washington, DC: American Public Health Association, 1990.

QUASI-EXPERIMENT A situation in which the investigator lacks full control over the allocation and/or timing of intervention but nonetheless conducts the study as if it were an experiment, allocating subjects to groups. Inability to allocate subjects randomly is a common situation that may be best described as a quasi-experiment. See also NATURAL EXPERIMENT.

QUESTIONNAIRE A predetermined set of questions used to collect data—clinical data, social status, occupational group, etc. This term is often applied to a self-completed survey instrument, as contrasted with an INTERVIEW SCHEDULE.

QUETELET'S INDEX See BODY MASS INDEX.

QUEUEING THEORY A mathematical discipline featuring models that analyze the flow of people through a service or their use of resources and that attempts to optimize utilization.

"QUICK AND DIRTY" METHOD A method that yields a result rapidly but not necessarily with scientific rigor or validity. At least one variety, RAPID EPIDEMIOLOGIC ASSESSMENT, has great value and is not necessarily "dirty" (i.e., unreliable).

QUOTA SAMPLING A method by which the proportions in the sample in various subgroups (according to criteria such as age, sex, and social status of the individuals to be selected) are chosen to agree with the corresponding proportions in the population. The resulting sample may not be representative of characteristics that have not been taken into account.

QUOTIENT The result of the division of a numerator by a denominator.

R

RACE Persons who are relatively homogeneous with respect to biological inheritance. In a time of political correctness, classifying by race is done cautiously,[1,2] although some organizations, e.g., the American Public Health Association, ask members to record their racial/ethnic group on membership forms. Epidemiologic studies have, of course, helped to identify racial correlates of certain conditions and to dissect race from socioeconomic and environmental conditions as determinants of disease. In Australia, the word *Europid* is sometimes used to describe persons of European origin, e.g., in multiethnic studies of diabetes and hypertension.

See also ETHNIC GROUP.

[1] Cooper R, David R. The biological concept of race and its application to public health and epidemiology. *J Health Polit Policy Law* 1986; II(1):97–116.
[2] Osborne NG, Feit MD. The use of race in medical research. *JAMA* 1992; 267:275–279.

RADIX The hypothetical size of the birth cohort in a life table, commonly 1000 or 100,000.

RAHE-HOLMES SOCIAL READJUSTMENT RATING SCALE See LIFE EVENTS.

RANDOM Governed by chance; not completely determined by other factors. As opposed to deterministic.

RANDOM-ACCESS MEMORY (RAM) Computer storage in which an arbitrary ("random") data unit can be read or a new data unit entered in its place, i.e., the memory storage is temporary.

RANDOM ALLOCATION, RANDOMIZATION Allocation of individuals to groups, e.g., for experimental and control regimens, by chance. Within the limits of chance variation, random allocation should make the control and experimental groups similar at the start of an investigation and ensure that personal judgment and prejudices of the investigator do not influence allocation.

Random allocation should not be confused with haphazard assignment. Random allocation follows a predetermined plan that is usually devised with the aid of a table of random numbers. The pattern of allocation may appear to be haphazard, but this arises from the haphazard nature with which digits occur in a table of random numbers, and not from the haphazard whim of the investigator in allocating patients.

RANDOM-DIGIT DIALING A method for sampling people in telephone surveys in which telephone numbers are randomly dialed.

RANDOM WALK The path traversed by a particle that moves in steps, each step being determined by chance in regard to direction, magnitude, or both. The theory of random walks has many applications, e.g., to sequential sampling and to the migration of insects, including disease vectors.

RANDOMIZED CONTROLLED TRIAL (RCT) An epidemiologic experiment in which subjects in a population are randomly allocated into groups, usually called *study* and *control* groups, to receive or not to receive an experimental preventive or therapeutic procedure, maneuver, or intervention. The results are assessed by rigorous comparison of rates of disease, death, recovery, or other appropriate outcome in the study and control groups, respectively. Randomized controlled trials are generally regarded as the most scientifically rigorous method of hypothesis testing available in epidemiology. A few authors refer to this method as "randomized control trial." See also EXPERIMENTAL EPIDEMIOLOGY.

RANDOM SAMPLE A sample that is arrived at by selecting sample units such that each possible unit has a fixed and determinate probability of selection. See also SAMPLE.

RANGE OF DISTRIBUTION The difference between the largest and smallest values in a distribution.

RANKING SCALE (ordinal scale) A scale that arrays the members of a group from high to low according to the magnitude of the observations, assigns numbers to the ranks, and neglects distances between members of the array.

RAPID EPIDEMIOLOGIC ASSESSMENT Methods that can be used to yield results as rapidly and efficiently as available resources permit, e.g., to assess health problems and evaluate health programs in developing countries or to delineate the health impact of a public health emergency such as a disaster or an epidemic with unusual features.[1]

[1] Rapid epidemiological assessment *Int J Epidemiol* 1989; 18 (Suppl 2):S1–S67.

RATE A rate is a measure of the frequency of occurrence of a phenomenon. In epidemiology, demography, and vital statistics, a rate is an expression of the frequency with which an event occurs in a defined population; the use of rates rather than raw numbers is essential for comparison of experience between populations at different times, different places, or among different classes of persons.

The components of a rate are the numerator, the denominator, the specified time in which events occur, and usually a multiplier, a power of 10, which converts the rate from an awkward fraction or decimal to a whole number:

$$\text{Rate} = \frac{\text{Number of events in specified period}}{\text{Average population during the period}} \times 10^n$$

All rates are ratios, calculated by dividing a numerator, e.g., the number of deaths, or newly occurring cases of a disease in a given period, by a denominator, e.g., the average population during that period. Some rates are proportions, i.e., the numerator is contained within the denominator. Rate has several different usages in epidemiology.

1. As a synonym for ratio, it refers to proportions as rates, as in the terms cumulative incidence rate, prevalence rate, survival rate (cf. *Webster's Third New International Dictionary,* which gives proportion and ratio as synonyms for rate).
2. In other situations, rate refers only to ratios representing relative changes (actual or potential) in two quantities. This accords with the *OED,* which gives "relative amount of variation" among its entries for rate.
3. Sometimes rate is further restricted to refer only to ratios representing changes over time. In this usage, prevalence rate would not be a "true" rate because it cannot be expressed in relation to units of time but only to a "point" in time; in contrast, the force of mortality or force of morbidity (hazard rate) is a "true" rate for it can be expressed as the number of cases developing per unit time, divided by the total size of the population at risk.

RATE DIFFERENCE (RD) The absolute difference between two rates, for example, the difference in incidence rate between a population group exposed to a causal factor and a population group not exposed to the factor:

$$RD = I_e - I_u$$

where I_e = incidence rate among exposed, and I_u = incidence rate among unexposed. In comparisons of exposed and unexposed groups, the term *excess rate* may be used as a synonym for *rate difference*.

RATE-ODDS RATIO See ODDS RATIO.

RATE RATIO (RR) The ratio of two rates. The term is used in epidemiologic research with a precise meaning, i.e., the ratio of the rate in the exposed population to the rate in the unexposed population:

$$RR = \frac{I_e}{I_u}$$

where I_e is the incidence rate among exposed, and I_u is the incidence rate among unexposed. See also RELATIVE RISK.

RATIO The value obtained by dividing one quantity by another: a general term of which rate, proportion, percentage, etc., are subsets. The important difference between a proportion and a ratio is that the numerator of a proportion is included in the population defined by the denominator, whereas this is not necessarily so for a ratio. A ratio is an expression of the relationship between a numerator and a denominator where the two usually are separate and distinct quantities, neither being included in the other.

The dimensionality of a ratio is obtained through algebraic cancellation, summation, etc., of the dimensionalities of its numerator and denominator terms. Both counted and measured values may be included in the numerator and in the denominator. There are no general restrictions on the dimensionalities or ranges of ratios, as there are in some of its subsets (e.g., proportion, prevalence). Ratios are sometimes expressed as percentages (e.g., standardized mortality ratio, FEV_1 percent). In these cases, unlike the special case of a PROPORTION, the value may exceed 100. See also PROPORTION; RATE.

RATIO SCALE See MEASUREMENT SCALE.

RAW DATA The entire set of information that has been collected in a study, before any cleaning, editing or statistical manipulation begins.

READ-ONLY MEMORY (ROM) Computer storage that does not allow modification of its contents, i.e., storage is permanent.

REASON FOR ENCOUNTER (RFE) The statement of reason(s) why a person enters the health care system, representing that person's demand for care. The terms recorded by the health care provider clarify the reason for encounter without interpreting it in the form of a diagnosis.[1]

[1] Lamberts H, Wood M. *ICPC, International Classification of Primary Care*. New York: Oxford University Press, 1987.

RECALL BIAS Systematic error due to differences in accuracy or completeness of recall to memory of past events or experiences. For example, a mother whose child has died of leukemia is more likely than the mother of a healthy living child to remember details of such past experiences as use of x-ray services when the child was in utero.

RECEIVER OPERATING CHARACTERISTIC (ROC) CURVE (Syn: relative operating characteristic curve) A graphic means for assessing the ability of a screening test to discriminate between healthy and diseased persons. The term *receiver operating characteristic* comes from psychometry, where the characteristic operating response of a receiver-individual to faint stimuli or nonstimuli was recorded.

RECESSIVE In genetics, a gene that is phenotypically manifest only when present in the homozygous state.

RECOMMENDATIONS See GUIDELINES.

RECORD LINKAGE A method for assembling the information contained in two or more records—e.g., in different sets of medical charts, and in vital records such as birth and death certificates—and a procedure to ensure that the same individual is counted only once. This procedure incorporates a unique identifying system such as a personal identification number and/or birth name(s) of the individual's mother.[1]

Record linkage makes it possible to relate significant health events that are remote from one another in time and place or to bring together records of different individuals, e.g., members of a family. The resulting information is generally stored and retrieved by computer, which can be programmed to tabulate and analyze the data.

Each person in the world creates a book of life. This book starts with birth and ends with death. Its pages are made of the records of the principal events in life. Record linkage is the name given to the process of assembling the pages of this book into a volume.[2]

[1] Newcombe HB. *Handbook of Record Linkage*. Oxford, England: Oxford Medical Publications, 1988.
[2] Dunn HL: Record linkage. *Am J Public Health* 1946; 36:1412.

RECRUDESCENCE Reactivation of infection.

RECTANGULARIZATION OF MORTALITY The shape of the graph as life expectancy increases: higher proportions of all who are born survive to old age and the graph becomes more "rectangular" in shape.[1] Empirical observations in several countries have failed to demonstrate it. Olshansky[2] found the opposite happening in the USA—the range of age at death is widening because of the impact of HIV disease and violence.

[1] Fries JF. Aging, natural death, and the compression of morbidity. *N Engl J Med* 1980; 303:130–135.
[2] Olshansky SJ, Carnes BA, Cassel C: In search of Methuselah: estimating the upper limits of human longevity. *Science* 1990; 250:634–640.

REDEFINING THE UNACCEPTABLE An expression used by Vickers[1] to describe the history of public health. The public health advances when there is a combination of knowledge of the causes of public health problems, technical capability to deal with these causes, a sense of values that the health problems are important, and political will. It is the last of these that Vickers described as "redefining the unacceptable."

[1] Vickers GR. What sets the goals of public health? *Lancet* 1958; 1:599–604.

REDUCTION (of data)

1. (Syn: "collapsing") Reducing the number of categories of a set of data to simplify analysis. An important application is aggregation of small numbers and/or small areas in published tables from a national census in order to preserve the CONFIDENTIALITY of these localities and their residents.
2. Formation of composite (derived) variables based on several originally collected variables, using methods ranging from simple indices to factor analysis.

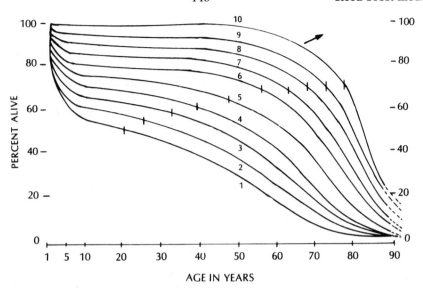

1. India, Male, 1901-1911. (Expectation of life at birth, 22.59 years)
2. Guatemala, Male, 1921. (25.59 years)
3. Mexico, Male, 1930. (33.02 years)
4. England and Wales, Male, 1861. (40.47 years)
5. Guatemala, Male, 1964. (48.51 years)
6. England and Wales, Male, 1921. (55.94 years)
7. Venezuela, Male, 1964. (63.74 years)
8. Netherlands, Male, 1947-49. (69.40 years)
9. Sweden, Male, 1964. (75.93 years)
10. Sweden, Female, 1974. (78.10 years)

Rectangularization of mortality. Survivorship curves by age and sex, selected countries, 1861–1974. Vertical bars show life expectancy at birth. From Basch PF: *Textbook of International Health.* New York: Oxford University Press, 1990. With permission.

  3. Summarizing data by means of classification schemes and arithmetical manipulations.

REDUCTIONISM The idea that scientific disciplines can be united, e.g., by reducing psychology to physiology, physiology to chemistry, chemistry to physics, etc., and efforts and attitudes derived from this idea.

REED-FROST MODEL A mathematical model of infectious disease transmission and herd immunity developed by Lowell Reed and Wade Hampton Frost (1880–1938). The model gives the number of new cases, C, of an infectious disease that can be expected in a closed, freely mixing population of immunes and susceptibles in time period t to $t + 1$, with varying assumptions about the distribution of each in the population:

$$C_{t+1} = S_t [1 - (1 - p)_t^c]$$

where C_{t+1} is the number of cases between time t and $t + 1$, S_t is the number of susceptibles at time t, and p is the probability that any specified individual will have contact with any other specified individual in the population. Elaborations of the model by Fox et al[1] provide the theoretical basis for immunization programs that control infectious diseases without necessarily achieving 100% immunization coverage.

[1] Fox JP, Elveback L, Scott, W et al. Herd immunity: Basic concept and relevance to public health immunization practices. *Am J Epidemiol* 1971; 94:179–189.

REFERENCE POPULATION The standard against which a population that is being studied can be compared.

REFINEMENT The process of identifying new subcategories of study variables for the purpose of more accurate or more detailed description of relationships. An example is refinement of the concept of serum cholesterol level into high, low, and very low density lipoproteins.

REGISTER, REGISTRY In epidemiology the term *register* is applied to the file of data concerning all cases of a particular disease or other health-relevant condition in a defined population such that the cases can be related to a population base. With this information, incidence rates can be calculated. If the cases are regularly followed up, information on remission, exacerbation, prevalence, and survival can also be obtained. The *register* is the actual document, and the *registry* is the system of ongoing registration.

In most developed countries all births and deaths are recorded through birth and death registration systems. Results and summaries are then tabulated and published. Examples of registries that have epidemiologic value include the following:

Cancer registries, which secure reports of cancer patients as soon as possible after first diagnosis. The principal sources for these reports are the hospitals serving the community, but a few cases are not reported until death.

Twin registries, which have provided the basis for studies attempting to differentiate genetic from environmental factors in the etiology of cancer and other conditions where both genetic and environmental factors may be contributing causes.

Birth defect registries, which seek to document anomalies that are apparent at or soon after birth. They suffer from incompleteness due to omission of stillbirths and of anomalies that do not declare their presence until later in life, such as certain forms of congenital heart lesion, mental deficiency, and neurological disorders.

Many types of register—e.g., disease-specific, treatment-specific, "at risk," local (hospital- or clinic-based)—are not population-based. Population-based registers are usually considered to be the most useful type for epidemiologic purposes; clinic-based, disease-specific registers can be used as a source of cases for case control studies.[1]

[1] Goldberg J, Gelfand HM, Levy PS. Registry evaluation methods. *Epidemiol Rev* 1980; 2:210–220.

REGISTRATION The term *registration* implies something more than notification for the purpose of immediate action or to permit the counting of cases. A register requires that a permanent record be established, including identifying data. Cases may be followed up, and statistical tabulations may be prepared both on frequency and on survival. In addition, the persons listed on a register may be subjects of special studies.

REGRESSION

1. As used by Francis Galton (1822–1911), one of the founders of modern biology and biometry, in his book *Hereditary Genius* (1869), this meant the tendency of offspring of exceptional parents (unusually tall, unusually intelligent, etc.) to possess characteristics closer to the average for the general population. Hence "regression to the mean."

2. In statistics, regression is a synonym for REGRESSION ANALYSIS.

REGRESSION ANALYSIS Given data on a dependent variable y and one or more independent variables x_1, x_2, etc., regression analysis involves finding the "best" mathematical model (within some restricted class of models) to describe y as a function of the x's, or to predict y from the x's. The most common form is a linear model; in epidemiology, the logistic and proportional hazards models are also common.

REGRESSION LINE Diagrammatic presentation of a regression equation, usually drawn with the independent variable, x, as the abscissa and the dependent variable, y, as ordinate. Three variables can be shown diagrammatically on an isometric chart or stereogram.

RELATIONSHIP See ASSOCIATION.

RELATIVE ODDS See ODDS RATIO.

RELATIVE RISK
1. The ratio of the RISK of disease or death among the exposed to the risk among the unexposed; this usage is synonymous with RISK RATIO.
2. Alternatively, the ratio of the cumulative incidence rate in the exposed to the cumulative incidence rate in the unexposed, i.e., the cumulative incidence ratio.
3. The term *relative risk* has also been used synonymously with *odds ratio* and, in some biostatistical articles, has been used for the ratio of FORCES OF MORBIDITY. The use of the term *relative risk* for several different quantities arises from the fact that for "rare" diseases (e.g., most cancers) all the quantities approximate one another. For common occurrences (e.g., neonatal mortality in infants under 1500-g birth weight), the approximations do not hold.

See also CUMULATIVE INCIDENCE RATIO; ODDS RATIO; RATE RATIO; RISK RATIO.

RELIABILITY The degree of stability exhibited when a measurement is repeated under identical conditions. *Reliability* refers to the degree to which the results obtained by a measurement procedure can be replicated. Lack of reliability may arise from divergences between observers or instruments of measurement or instability of the attribute being measured. See also MEASUREMENT, TERMINOLOGY OF; OBSERVER VARIATION.

REPEATABILITY (Syn: reproducibility) A test or measurement is repeatable if the results are identical or closely similar each time it is conducted. See also MEASUREMENT, TERMINOLOGY OF; RELIABILITY.

REPLACEMENT LEVEL FERTILITY The level of fertility at which a cohort of women are having only enough daughters to replace themselves in the population. By definition, replacement-level fertility is equal to a net reproduction rate of 1.00. The total fertility rate is also used as a measure of replacement-level fertility; in the United States today, a total fertility rate of 2.12 is considered to be replacement level; it is higher than 2 because of mortality and because of a sex ratio greater than 1 at birth. The higher the female mortality rate, the higher is replacement-level fertility.

REPLICATION The execution of an experiment or survey more than once so as to confirm the findings, increase precision, and obtain a closer estimation of sampling error. *Exact replication* should be distinguished from *consistency of results on replication*. Exact replication is often possible in the physical sciences, but in the biological and behavioral sciences, to which epidemiology belongs, consistency of results on replication is often the best that can be attained. Consistency of results on replication is perhaps the most important criterion in judgments of causality.

REPORTING BIAS Selective revealing or suppression of information about past medical history, e.g., details of sexual experiences.

REPRESENTATIVE SAMPLE The term *representative* as it is commonly used is undefined in the statistical or mathematical sense; it means simply that the sample resembles the population in some way.

The use of probability sampling will not ensure that any single sample will be "representative" of the population in all possible respects. If, for example, it is found that the sample age distribution is quite different from that of the population, it is possible to make corrections for the known differences. A common fallacy lies in the unwarranted assumption that, if the sample resembles the population closely on those factors that have been checked, it is "totally representative" and that no difference exists between the sample and the universe or reference population.

Kendall and Buckland[1] comment as follows: "In the widest sense, a sample which is representative of a population. Some confusion arises according to whether 'representative' is regarded as meaning 'selected by some process which gives all samples an equal chance of appearing to represent the population'; or, alternatively, whether it means 'typical in respect of certain characteristics, however chosen'. On the whole, it seems best to confine the word 'representative' to samples which turn out to be so, however chosen, rather than apply it to those chosen with the object of being representative."

[1] Kendall MG, Buckland WR. *A Dictionary of Statistical Terms,* 4th ed. London: Longman, 1982.

REPRODUCIBILITY See REPEATABILITY.

REPRODUCTIVE ISOLATION Absence of interbreeding between populations.

REPRODUCTIVE SUCCESS In population genetics, quantitatively, the proportion of offspring surviving long enough to reproduce.

RESEARCH The organized quest for new knowledge, based on curiosity or on perceived needs. Research may consist of systematic empirical observation or hypothesis testing and the use of a preplanned research design such as an EXPERIMENT.

RESEARCH DESIGN The procedures and methods, predetermined by an investigator, to be adhered to in conducting a research project.

RESEARCH ETHICS BOARD, COMMITTEE See INSTITUTIONAL REVIEW BOARD.

RESERVOIR OF INFECTION
1. Any person, animal, arthropod, plant, soil, or substance, or a combination of these, in which an infectious agent normally lives and multiplies, on which it depends primarily for survival, and where it reproduces itself in such a manner that it can be transmitted to a susceptible host.
2. The natural habitat of the infectious agent.

RESIDUAL CONFOUNDING Potential confounding by factors or variables not yet considered in the analysis; these may be directly observable or not; in the latter case, they are latent residual confounders.

RESOLUTION, RESOLVING POWER
1. The capacity of a system to distinguish between truly distinct things that are close together.
2. A component of a measuring instrument that helps determine precision. The degree of refinement of the measuring process is commonly referred to as the "resolution" or the "resolving power of the system." See also POWER. The capability of distinguishing between things that are indeed separate or distinct from one another.

RESOURCE ALLOCATION The process of deciding how to distribute financial, material, and human resources among competing claimants for these resources. Resource allocation is an essential feature of all health planning everywhere. Epidemiologic evidence on need, demand, supply, and use of existing services is integral to the process, although pragmatic factors such as political and emotional considerations sometimes carry more weight than objective epidemiologic evidence; on the other hand, ethical considerations seldom affect decisions about resource allocation.

RESPONSE BIAS Systematic error due to differences in characteristics between those who choose or volunteer to take part in a study and those who do not.

RESPONSE RATE The number of completed or returned survey instruments (questionnaires, interviews, etc.) divided by the total number of persons who would have been surveyed if all had participated. Usually expressed as a percentage. Nonresponse can have several causes, e.g., death, removal out of the survey community, and refusal. See also BIAS; COMPLETION RATE; NONPARTICIPANTS.

RETROLECTIVE Pertaining to data gathered from medical records or other sources, when data collection took place without prior planning for the needs of an investigation. See also PROLECTIVE; a term suggested by A. R. Feinstein.[1]

[1] Feinstein AR. Strategy of comparison in cause-effect research, in *Clinical Epidemiology*. Philadelphia: Saunders, 1985:215–236.

RETROSPECTIVE STUDY A research design that is used to test etiologic hypotheses in which inferences about exposure to the putative causal factor(s) are derived from data relating to characteristics of the persons under study or to events or experiences in their past. The essential feature is that some of the persons under study have the disease or other outcome condition of interest, and their characteristics and past experiences are compared with those of other, unaffected persons. Persons who differ in the severity of the disease may also be compared. There is disagreement among epidemiologists as to the desirability of using the term *retrospective study* rather than *case control study* to describe this method. See also CASE CONTROL STUDY.

RETROVIRUS This name is given to a family of RNA viruses characterized by the presence of an enzyme, reverse transcriptase, that enables transcription of RNA to DNA inside an affected cell. Thus, retroviruses can make copies of themselves in host cells. The most important retrovirus is the human immunodeficiency virus (HIV); this makes copies of itself in host cells such as T4 "helper" lymphocytes and normal immune responses are disrupted.

REVERSE TRANSCRIPTION The process by which an RNA molecule is used as a template to make a single-stranded DNA copy. This is the mode of action of the HUMAN IMMUNODEFICIENCY VIRUS when it attacks T4 helper lymphocytes, which maintain immune competence.

RIDIT A method of presenting observed values, e.g., health measurement scale scores of a group, relative to a reference population.[1] The average ridit for the group shows the probability that a member of the group differs from a member of the reference population. For example, if the average ridit for a group is 0.62, 62% of persons in the reference population have higher scores than a randomly chosen member of the group.

[1] Patrick DL, Erickson P. *Health Status and Health Policy: Allocating Resources to Health Care.* New York: Oxford University Press, 1993.

RIDIT ANALYSIS A method proposed by Bross (1958) for analyzing subjectively categorized or poorly recorded data. It consists of allocating scores relative to the identified distribution of the data based upon a transformation to the uniform distribution rather than the normal distribution.

RISK The probability that an event will occur, e.g., that an individual will become ill or die within a stated period of time or age. Also, a nontechnical term encompassing a variety of measures of the probability of a (generally) unfavorable outcome. See also PROBABILITY.

RISK ASSESSMENT The qualitative or quantitative estimation of the likelihood of adverse effects that may result from exposure to specified health hazards or from the absence of beneficial influences.

RISK ASSESSMENT The process of determining risks to health attributable to environmental or other hazards.[1] The process consists of four steps, as follows:

1. *Hazard identification:* Identifying the agent responsible for the health problem, its adverse effects, the target population, and the conditions of exposure.
2. *Risk characterization:* Describing the potential health effects of the hazard, quantifying dose-effect and dose-response relationships.
3. *Exposure assessment:* Quantifying exposure (dose) in a specified population, based on measurement of emissions, environmental levels of toxic substances, biologic monitoring, etc.
4. *Risk estimation:* Combining risk characterization, dose-response relationships and exposure estimates to quantify the risk level in a specific population. The end result is a qualitative and quantitative statement about the health effects expected and the proportion and number of affected people in a target population, including estimates of the uncertainties involved. The size of the exposed population must be known.

[1] *Assessment and Management of Environmental Health Hazards.* Geneva: WHO (mimeograph; WHO/PEP/89.6).

RISK-BENEFIT ANALYSIS The process of analyzing and comparing on a single scale the expected positive (benefits) and negative (risks, costs) results of an action, or lack of an action.

RISK-BENEFIT RATIO The results of a risk benefit analysis, expressed as the ratio of risks to benefits.

RISK CHARACTERIZATION See RISK ASSESSMENT

RISK DIFFERENCE (Syn: excess risk) The absolute difference between two risks.

RISK ESTIMATION See RISK ASSESSMENT

RISK EVALUATION See RISK MANAGEMENT

RISK FACTOR An aspect of personal behavior or life-style, an environmental exposure, or an inborn or inherited characteristic, which on the basis of epidemiologic evidence is known to be associated with health-related condition(s) considered important to prevent. The term *risk factor* is rather loosely used, with any of the following meanings:

1. An attribute or exposure that is associated with an increased probability of a specified outcome, such as the occurrence of a disease. Not necessarily a causal factor. A RISK MARKER.
2. An attribute or exposure that increases the probability of occurrence of disease or other specified outcome. A DETERMINANT.
3. A determinant that can be modified by intervention, thereby reducing the probability of occurrence of disease or other specified outcomes. To avoid confusion, it may be referred to as a modifiable risk factor.

The term *risk factor* became popular after its frequent use by T. R. Dawber and others in papers from the Framingham study published in and after 1961.

RISK MANAGEMENT The steps taken to alter, i.e., reduce, the levels of risk to which an individual or a population is subject. The managerial, decision-making and active hazard control process to deal with environmental agents of disease such as toxic substances for which risk evaluation has indicated an unacceptably high level of risk.[1] The process consists of three steps, as follows:

1. *Risk evaluation:* Comparison of calculated risks, or public health impact, of exposure to an environmental agent with the risks caused by other agents or societal factors, and with the benefits associated with the agent, as a basis for deciding what is an ACCEPTABLE RISK.

2. *Exposure control:* Actions taken to keep exposure below an acceptable maximum limit.

3. *Risk monitoring:* The process of measuring reduction in risk after exposure control actions have been taken, in order to reassess risks and initiate further control measures if necessary.

[1] *Assessment and Management of Environmental Health Hazards.* Geneva: WHO (mimeograph; WHO/PEP/89.6).

RISK MARKER (Syn: risk indicator) An attribute that is associated with an increased probability of occurrence of a disease or other specified outcome and that can be used as an indicator of this increased risk. Not necessarily a causal factor. See also RISK FACTOR.

RISK RATIO The ratio of two risks.

ROBUST A statistical test or procedure is said to be robust if it is not very sensitive to departures from the assumptions on which it is strictly predicted (e.g., that the data are normally distributed).

ROUNDING The process of eliminating surplus digits, taking the nearest whole number, multiple of 10, etc., as an approximation of the value of a measurement. See also DIGIT PREFERENCE.

RUBRIC Section or chapter heading. Used in epidemiology with reference to groups of diseases, e.g., as in the INTERNATIONAL CLASSIFICATION OF DISEASE (ICD).

S

SAFETY FACTOR A multiplicative factor incorporated in risk assessments or safety standards to allow for unpredictable types of variation, such as variability from test animals to humans, random variation within an experiment, and person-to-person variability. Safety factors are often in the range of 10 to 1000 or even higher magnitudes.

SAFETY STANDARDS Under the requirements of the Occupational Safety and Health Act (OSHA, 1970), *occupational safety and health standard* means a standard that requires conditions, or the adoption of one or more practices, means, methods, operations, or processes reasonably necessary or appropriate to provide safe or healthful employment and places of employment. Safety standards may be adopted by national consensus or established by federal regulation. These standards have been adopted in many other nations besides the United States, although some European and other countries have their own standards, which may be either more or less stringent than those in the United States.

There are several varieties of safety standards:
1. OSHA-promulgated, mainly for carcinogens, also for cotton dust and lead. These are *Permissable Exposure Limits* (PELs).
2. National Institute of Occupational Safety and Health (NIOSH) recommendations, often lower limits, based on animal toxicity tests, empirical observations, epidemiologic investigations; these are *Recommended Exposure Limits* (RELs).
3. An older-established set of criteria has been set by the American Conference of Governmental Industrial Hygienists; these are *Threshhold Limit Values* (TLVs) that have replaced an earlier set of Maximum Allowable Concentrations (MACs).

SAMPLE A selected subset of a population. A sample may be random or nonrandom and may be representative or nonrepresentative. Several types of sample can be distinguished, including the following:

Area sample: See AREA SAMPLING.

Cluster sample: Each unit selected is a group of persons (all persons in a city block, a family, etc.) rather than an individual.

Grab sample (Syn: sample of convenience): These ill-defined terms describe samples selected by easily employed but basically nonprobabilistic methods. "Man-in-the-street" surveys and a survey of blood pressure among volunteers who drop in at an examination booth in a public place are in this category. It is improper to generalize from the results of a survey based upon such a sample for there is no way of knowing what sorts of bias may have been operating. See also BIAS.

Probability (random) sample: All individuals have a known chance of selection. They may all have an equal chance of being selected, or, if a stratified sampling method is used, the rate at which individuals from several subsets are sampled can be varied so as to produce greater representation of some classes than of others.

A probability sample is created by assigning an identity (label, number) to all individuals in the "universe" population, e.g., by arranging them in alphabetical order and numbering in sequence, or simply assigning a number to each, or by grouping according to area of residence and numbering the groups. The next step is to select individuals (or groups) for study by a procedure such as use of a table of random numbers (or comparable procedure) to ensure that the chance of selection is known.

Simple random sample: In this elementary kind of sample each person has an equal chance of being selected out of the entire population. One way of carrying out this procedure is to assign each person a number, starting with 1, 2, 3, and so on. Then numbers are selected at random, preferably from a table of random numbers, until the desired sample size is attained.

Stratified random sample: This involves dividing the population into distinct subgroups according to some important characteristic, such as age or socioeconomic status, and selecting a random sample out of each subgroup. If the proportion of the sample drawn from each of the subgroups, or strata, is the same as the proportion of the total population contained in each stratum (e.g., age group 40–59 constitutes 20% of the population, and 20% of the sample comes from this age stratum), then all strata will be fairly represented with regard to numbers of persons in the sample.

Systematic sample: The procedure of selecting according to some simple, systematic rule, such as all persons whose names begin with specified alphabetic letters, born on certain dates, or located at specified points on a master list. A systematic sample may lead to errors that invalidate generalizations. For example, persons' names more often begin with certain letters of the alphabet than with other letters, e.g., q, x. A systematic alphabetical sample is therefore likely to be biased.

SAMPLE, EPSEM ("equal probability of selection method") A sample selected in such a manner that all the population units have the same probability of selection. A simple random sample is an Epsem sample; a stratified sample is not unless the probability of selection is the same for all strata.

SAMPLE SIZE DETERMINATION The mathematical process of deciding, before a study begins, how many subjects should be studied. The factors to be taken into account include the incidence or prevalence of the condition being studied, the estimated or putative relationship among the variables in the study, the POWER that is desired, and the allowable magnitude of type I error.

SAMPLING The process of selecting a number of subjects from all the subjects in a particular group or "universe." Conclusions based on sample results may be attributed only to the population sampled. Any extrapolation to a larger or different population is a judgment or a guess and is not part of statistical inference.

SAMPLING BIAS Systematic error due to study of a nonrandom sample of a population.

SAMPLING ERROR That part of the total estimation error of a parameter caused by the random nature of the sample.

SAMPLING VARIATION Since the inclusion of individuals in a sample is determined by chance, the results of analysis in two or more samples will differ, purely by chance. This is known as "sampling variation."

SANITARY CORDON See CORDON SANITAIRE.

SARTWELL'S INCUBATION MODEL Philip Sartwell (1908–   ) showed that the incubation periods for communicable diseases have a log-normal distribution and that the incubation periods for certain cancers that have well-defined external causes also have a log-normal distribution.[1]

[1]Sartwell PE. The incubation period of infectious diseases. *Am J Hygiene* 1950; 51:320–321.

SCALE A device or system for measuring equal portions. A logarithmic scale measures equal powers of 10. Many kinds of scale are used in medicine and epidemiology. From the French and Middle English *scale*, a ladder.

SCATTER DIAGRAM, PLOT (Syn: scattergram) A graphic method of displaying the distribution of two variables in relation to each other. The values for one variable are measured on the horizontal axis and the values for the other on the vertical axis.

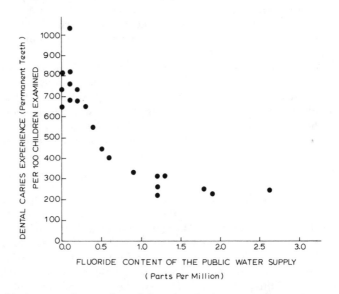

Relationship between the number of dental caries in permanent teeth and flouride content in the public water supply. From Lilienfeld and Stolley, 1994.

SCENARIO BUILDING A method of predicting the future that relies on a series of assumptions about alternative possibilities, rather than on simple extrapolation of existing trends.[1] Trend lines for demographic composition, morbidity and mortality rates, etc., can then be modified by allowing for each assumption in turn, or combinations of assumptions. The method is claimed to lead to greater flexibility in long-range health planning than simple forecasting that relies only upon extrapolation of trends.

[1]Brouwer JJ, Schreuder RF. *Scenarios and Other Methods to Support Long Term Health Planning.* Utrecht: Jan van Arkel, 1988.

SCIENTOMETRICS The measurement of scientific output and the impact of scientific findings, e.g., on public policy. This activity is sufficiently developed to have its own journal, *Scientometrics.*

SCREENING Screening was defined in 1951 by the US Commission on Chronic Illness as, "The presumptive identification of unrecognized disease or defect by the application of tests, examinations or other procedures which can be applied rapidly. Screening tests sort out apparently well persons who probably have a disease from those who probably do not. A screening test is not intended to be diagnostic. Persons with positive or suspicious findings must be referred to their physicians for diagnosis and necessary treatment."

Screening is an initial examination only, and positive responders require a second, diagnostic examination. The initiative for screening usually comes from the investigator or the person or agency providing care rather than from a patient with a complaint. Screening is usually concerned with chronic illness and aims to detect disease not yet under medical care.[1]

There are different types of medical screening, each with its own aim: mass, multiple or multiphasic, and prescriptive.

Mass screening simply means the screening of a whole population.

Multiple or multiphasic screening involves the use of a variety of screening tests on the same occasion.

Prescriptive screening has as its aim the early detection in presumptively healthy individuals of specific diseases that can be controlled better if detected early in their natural history.[2] An example is the use of mammography to detect breast cancer.

The characteristics of a screening test include accuracy, estimates of yield, precision, reproducibility, sensitivity and specificity, and validity. See entries under these headings.[3]

[1] Wilson JMG, Jungner G. *The Principles and Practice of Screening for Disease.* Geneva: WHO, 1968.
[2] *Guide to Clinical Preventive Services: Report of the US Preventive Services Task Force.* Baltimore: Williams & Wilkins, 1989.
[3] Morrison AS. *Screening in Chronic Disease,* 2nd ed. New York: Oxford University Press, 1993.

SCREENING LEVEL The normal limit or cutoff point at which a screening test is regarded as positive.

SEASONAL VARIATION Change in physiological status or in disease occurrence that conforms to a regular seasonal pattern.

SECONDARY ATTACK RATE The number of cases of an infection that occur among contacts within the incubation period following exposure to a primary case in relation to the total number of exposed contacts; the denominator is restricted to susceptible contacts when these can be determined. The secondary attack rate is a measure of contagiousness and is useful in evaluating control measures. See also ATTACK RATE, BASIC REPRODUCTIVE RATE.

SECTOR In the language used by UN agencies (WHO, UNICEF, etc.), a sector is a defined component of the body politic such as the health sector, the education sector, the housing sector.

SECULAR TREND (Syn: temporal trend) Changes over a long period of time, generally years or decades. Examples include the decline of tuberculosis mortality and the rise, followed by a decline, in coronary heart disease mortality in many industrial countries in the past 50 years.

SELECTION In genetics, the force that brings about changes in the frequency of alleles and genotypes in populations through differential reproduction. In epidemiology, the process and procedure for choosing individuals for study, usually by an orderly means such as random allocation.

SELECTION BIAS Error due to systematic differences in characteristics between those who are selected for study and those who are not. Examples include subjects in a survey limited to volunteers or persons present in a particular place at a particular time, or hospital cases under the care of a physician, excluding those who die before admission to hospital because the course of their disease is so acute, those not sick enough to require hospital care, or those excluded by cost, distance, or other factors. Selection bias invalidates conclusions and generalizations that might otherwise be drawn from such studies. It is a common and commonly overlooked problem.

SENSITIVITY ANALYSIS A method to determine the robustness of an assessment by examining the extent to which results are affected by changes in methods, values of variables, or assumptions. The aim is to identify variables whose values are most likely to change the results or to find a solution that is relatively stable for the most commonly occurring values of these variables.

SENSITIVITY AND SPECIFICITY (of a screening test) *Sensitivity* is the proportion of truly diseased persons in the screened population who are identified as diseased by the screening test. Sensitivity is a measure of the probability of correctly diagnosing a case, or the probability that any given case will be identified by the test (Syn: true positive rate).

Specificity is the proportion of truly nondiseased persons who are so identified by the screening test. It is a measure of the probability of correctly identifying a non-diseased person with a screening test (Syn: true negative rate). The relationships are shown in the following fourfold table, in which the letters *a*, *b*, *c*, and *d* represent the quantities specified below the table.

Screening test results	True status		TOTAL
	Diseased	Not diseased	
Positive	a	b	$a+b$
Negative	c	d	$c+d$
Total	$a+c$	$b+d$	$a+b+c+d$

a. Diseased individuals detected by the test (true positives)
b. Nondiseased individuals positive by the test (false positives)
c. Diseased individuals not detectable by the test (false negatives)
d. Nondiseased individuals negative by the test (true negatives)

$$\text{Sensitivity} = \frac{a}{a+c} \qquad \text{Specificity} = \frac{d}{b+d}$$

$$\text{Predictive value (positive test result)} = \frac{a}{a+b}$$

$$\text{Predictive value (negative test result)} = \frac{d}{c+d}$$

The predictive value of a positive test result is called the *yield*. See also YOUDEN'S INDEX.

SENSITIVITY TESTING A study of how the final outcome of an analysis changes as a function of varying one or more of the input parameters in a prescribed manner.

SENTINEL HEALTH EVENT A condition that can be used to assess the stability or change in health levels of a population, usually by monitoring mortality statistics. Thus, death due to acute head injury is a sentinel event for a class of severe traffic injury that may be reduced by such preventive measures as use of seat belts and crash helmets.

SENTINEL PHYSICIAN, SENTINEL PRACTICE In family medicine, a physician, practice, that undertakes to maintain surveillance for and report certain specific predetermined events, such as cases of certain communicable diseases, adverse drug reactions.

SEQUENTIAL ANALYSIS A statistical method that allows an experiment to be ended as soon as an answer of the desired precision is obtained. Study and control subjects are randomly allocated in pairs or blocks. The result of the comparison of each pair of subjects, one treated and one control, is examined as soon as it becomes available and is added to all previous results.

SERENDIPITY The accidental (and happy) discovery of important new information. A well-known example is Fleming's discovery of the bacteriocidal properties of penicillin mould. In case-control studies aimed at testing a specific hypothesis, e.g., about the relationship between tobacco and cancer, questions on other aspects of life-style have serendipitously revealed statistically significant associations, e.g., between alcohol consumption and certain cancers.

SERIAL INTERVAL (Syn: generation time) The period of time between analogous phases of an infectious illness in successive cases of a chain of infection that is spread person to person.

SEROEPIDEMIOLOGY Epidemiologic study or activity based on the detection on serological testing of characteristic change in the serum level of specific antibodies. Latent, subclinical infections and carrier states can thus be detected, in addition to clinically overt cases.

SET A defined group of events, objects, data, that is distinguishable from other groups.

SET THEORY Branch of mathematics and logic dealing with the characteristics and relationships of sets.

SEX RATIO The ratio of one sex to the other. Usually defined as the ratio of males to females (or of the rates observed in males and females).

SF36 Acronym for the 36-item questionnaire derived from the longer set of questions used in household interview surveys conducted by the US National Center for Health Statistics. The SF36 questions measure eight multi-item variables: physical function, social function, role limitation, mental health, energy, vitality, pain, and general perception of health. The instrument has been widely adopted, although some authors have raised doubts about its validity.

SHARPS A jargon term for any sharp-pointed object that has been used in a health care setting and that, if the sharp end is contaminated by pathogens and it pierces the skin, could convey infection to a health care worker or other person. Safe disposal of sharps has become increasingly important in hospital practice since the onset of the HIV epidemic.

"SHOE-LEATHER" EPIDEMIOLOGY Gathering information for epidemiologic studies by direct inquiry among the people, e.g., walking from door to door and asking questions of every householder (wearing out shoe leather in the process). John Snow (1813–1858) did this when investigating the sources of water supply to households in the cholera epidemic in London in 1854; the method has been successfully used in many subsequent epidemic investigations. It is especially useful in investigations of sexually transmitted diseases. Much of the work of the Epidemic Intelligence Service (EIS) is based on "shoe-leather epidemiology"; EIS officers have a club tie displaying the sole of a shoe with a hole in it, the result of wearing out much shoe leather in the course of their work.

SIBLINGS Children borne by the same mother.

SIBSHIP All the brothers and sisters borne by the same mother.

SICKNESS The state of dysfunction or the social role of a person with a DISEASE.

SIDE EFFECT An effect, other than the intended one, produced by a preventive, diagnostic, or therapeutic procedure or regimen. Not necessarily harmful.

SIDESTREAM SMOKE Smoke from combusted tobacco products, usually cigarettes, that is not filtered through the cigarette or the smoker's respiratory system but directly enters the air where its toxic and irritant effects on nonsmokers can lead to adverse health effects. See also ENVIRONMENTAL TOBACCO SMOKE.

SIGN TEST A test that can be used when combining results of several studies, e.g., in METAANALYSIS. The test considers the direction of results of individual studies, i.e., whether the associations demonstrated are positive or negative.

SIGNAL-TO-NOISE RATIO A jargon term for the relationship of pertinent findings to that which is extraneous or irrelevant, or intrudes because measurement methods or other procedures are insufficiently sensitive.

SIGNIFICANCE See STATISTICAL SIGNIFICANCE. Note the distinction between clinical and statistical significance; clinical significance is the more important. For example, when large numbers of comparisons are made, some differences will be "statistically significant" by chance; i.e., they are meaningless.

SIMPSON'S PARADOX A form of confounding, in which the presence of a confounding variable changes the direction of an association. Simpson's paradox can occur in METAANALYSIS, because the sum of the data or results from a number of different studies may be affected by confounding variables that have been excluded by design features from some studies but not others; if this is not recognized, meta-analysis will be flawed. Rothman[1] has pointed out that Simpson's paradox is not really a paradox but the logical consequence of failing to recognize the presence of confounding variables.

[1] Rothman KJ. A pictorial representation of confounding in epidemiologic studies. *J Chronic Dis* 1975; 28:101–108.

SIMULATION The use of a model system, e.g., a mathematical model or an animal model, to approximate the action of a real system, often used to study the properties of a real system.

SINGLE-PATIENT TRIAL See N-OF-ONE STUDY.

SITUATION ANALYSIS Study of a situation that may require improvement. This begins with a definition of the problem and an assessment or measurement of its extent, severity, causes, and impacts upon the community and is followed by appraisal of interactions between the system and its environment and evaluations of performance.

SKEW DISTRIBUTION An older and less recommended term for an asymmetrical frequency distribution. If a unimodal distribution has a longer tail extending toward lower values of the variate, it is said to have negative skewness; in the contrary case, positive skewness. See also LOG-NORMAL DISTRIBUTION.

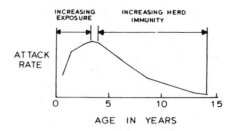

Skew distribution of attack rate of measles in relation to age.
From Lilienfeld and Stolley, 1994.

Skew diagram.

SLOW VIRUS Agent causing degenerative (neurological) diseases characterized by a long incubation period and a prolonged, slowly progressive course. The best-known confirmed slow virus diseases are Creutzfeldt-Jakob disease and kuru. Multiple sclerosis is possibly a slow virus disease. Some cases of HIV disease behave as slow virus disease. See also PRION.

SMOOTHING General term for methods of minimizing irregularities in a set of data. Examples include rounding, kriging, moving averages.

SNOWBALL SAMPLING A method of selecting for study the members of "hidden" populations, e.g., illicit drug users. Those initially identified are asked to name acquaintances who are added to the sample; these, in turn, are asked to name further acquaintances, and so on until enough numbers are accumulated to give adequate power to the proposed study. Compare CAPTURE-RECAPTURE METHOD.

SOCIAL CLASS A stratum in society composed of individuals and families of equal standing. See also SOCIOECONOMIC CLASSIFICATION.

SOCIAL DRIFT Downward social class mobility as a result of impaired health often due to mental disorders or substance abuse.

SOCIAL MARKETING The use of marketing theory, skills, and practice to achieve social change, e.g., in health promotion.

SOCIAL MEDICINE The practice of medicine concerned with health and disease as a function of group living. Social medicine is concerned with the health of people in relation to their behavior in social groups and as such involves care of the individual patient as a member of a family and of other significant groups in everyday life. It is also concerned with the health of these groups as such and with that of the whole community as a community. The "father of social medicine" is Johann Peter Frank (1745–1821) who described many features of this discipline in *System einer vollständigen medicinischen Polizey* (A System of Complete Medical Police, 1779). After the appointment of John Ryle (1889–1950) as the first professor of social medicine at the University of Oxford, this became the preferred term to describe academic departments dealing with this range of disciplines in the UK; in the 1970s the preferred term became COMMUNITY MEDICINE. The Acheson Report (1988) advocated the term PUBLIC HEALTH MEDICINE, which has been adopted by the Faculty of Community Medicine of the UK Royal Colleges of Physicians and many British academic departments. The frequent changes of terminology for the discipline contrast with the stability of terms such as anatomy and psychiatry, and unnerve those who fear that the process may be ongoing. See also COMMUNITY MEDICINE; PUBLIC HEALTH.

SOCIAL NETWORK INDEX A measure of the extent to which individuals or groups are connected to or isolated from others, i.e., family, friends and working colleagues. Health status has been found to be positively associated with the extent of social networks.[1]

[1] Berkman LF, Breslow L: *Health and Ways of Living: the Alameda County Study.* New York: Oxford University Press, 1983.

SOCIETAL RISK Probability of harm to the human population including probability of adverse health effects to descendants and probability of disruption resulting from loss of services such as industrial plant, loss of material goods, electricity.

SOCIOECONOMIC CLASSIFICATION Arrangement of persons into groups according to such characteristics as prior education, occupation, and income. This usually reveals upon analysis a strong correlation with health-related characteristics such as average length of life and risk of dying from certain specific causes.

The oldest such classification that is epidemiologically useful is the Registrar-General's (RG's) occupational classification, developed in 1911 by Stephenson, Registrar-General of England and Wales. This classified all occupations into five groups—the five "social classes." Social class III is often further subdivided into nonmanual and manual groups:

I Professional occupations
II Intermediate occupations
IIIN Nonmanual skilled occupations
IIIM Manual skilled occupations
IV Partly skilled occupations
V Unskilled occupations

This has proven to be a valuable epidemiologic tool; social class is a reliable and consistent predictor of health experience.

There have been many attempts to develop a more refined classification; however, most refinements require collection of more detailed information. For example, Hollingshead's scale requires details about education and income as well as occupation, and so is more time-consuming, more likely to be incomplete, and requires more costly analysis than the RG's classification. In developing countries, where up to 90% of the population may be classified under "agriculturalist" or "pastoralist" (farming or herding), other types of classifications have been developed.

One's prestige in society, and attitudes or values, e.g., setting a high value on getting a good education, are generally an integral part of social class or socioeconomic status. Attitudes toward health are often part of the set of values and may explain part of the observed difference in health between social classes.

SOCIOECONOMIC STATUS (SES) Descriptive term for a person's position in society, which may be expressed on an ORDINAL SCALE using such criteria as income, educational level attained, occupation, value of dwelling place, etc.

SOFTWARE See COMPUTER.

SOJOURN TIME (Syn: detectable preclinical period) The interval between detectability at screening and clinical presentation of a condition—i.e., the interval during which the condition is potentially detectable but not yet diagnosed[1]

[1] Alexander F. Estimation of sojourn time distributions and false negative rates in screening programmes which use two modalities. *Stat Med* 1989; 8:743–755.

SOUNDEX CODE A sequence of letters used for recording names phonetically, especially in RECORD LINKAGE.

SOURCE OF INFECTION The person, animal, object, or substance from which an infectious agent passes to a host. Source of infection should be clearly distinguished from source of contamination, such as overflow of a septic tank contaminating a water supply or an infected cook contaminating a salad. (See RESERVOIR OF INFECTION)[1]

[1] From Benenson AS, ed. *Control of Communicable Disease in Man,* 15th ed. Washington DC: American Public Health Association, 1990.

SPEARMAN'S RANK CORRELATION See CORRELATION COEFFICIENT.

SPECIFICATION

1. The process of selecting a particular functional form or model for the relationships to be analyzed in a study.
2. The process of selecting variables for inclusion in the analysis of an effect or association. This process leads to the identification of MODERATOR VARIABLES and CONFOUNDING VARIABLES. See also STRATIFICATION.

SPECIFICITY (OF A TEST) See SENSITIVITY AND SPECIFICITY.

SPECTRUM OF DISEASE The full range of manifestations of a disease; a vague term, which can mean everything from mild or subclinical or precursor states to fulminating, florid disease, or, alternatively, the natural history of a disease from onset to resolution.

SPELL OF SICKNESS An episode of sickness with a well-defined onset and termination. As used in the monitoring or surveillance of disease, the spell is often defined by the duration of absence from work or school.

SPLEEN RATE A term used in malaria epidemiology to define the frequency of enlarged spleens detected on survey of a population in which malaria is prevalent. In association with the HACKETT SPLEEN CLASSIFICATION, it summarizes the severity of malaria endemicity.

SPORADIC Occurring irregularly, haphazardly from time to time, and generally infrequently, e.g., cases of certain infectious diseases.

SPOT MAP Map showing the geographic location of people with a specific attribute, e.g., cases of a disease or elderly persons living alone. The making of a spot map is a common procedure in the investigation of a localized outbreak of disease. Inferences from such a map depend on the assumption that the population at risk of developing the disease is fairly evenly distributed over the area, or that at least the heterogeneities are known and can be considered in interpreting the map. A refinement is to indicate multiple cases at a single location by a series of short horizontal bars, as John Snow did to mark the location of cases of cholera in the epidemic in London in 1849; the method has been used by innumerable field epidemiologists ever since.

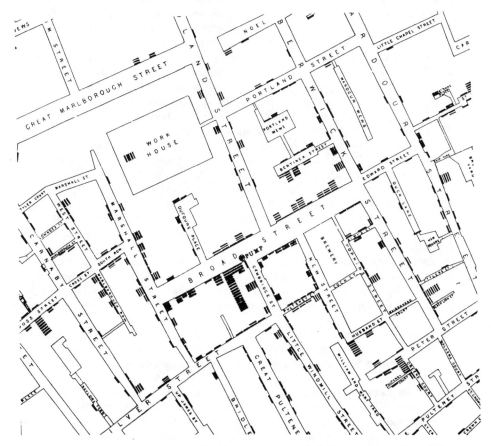

Spot map. From Snow, J: *On the Mode of Communication of Cholera.* London: Churchill, 1855.

SPREADSHEET A computer matrix of columns and rows in which numerical entries can be made on screen, stored, systematically manipulated, and modified.

STABLE POPULATION A population that has constant fertility and mortality rates, no migration, and consequently a fixed age distribution and constant growth rate. See also STATIONARY POPULATION.

STANDARD Something that serves as a basis for comparison; a technical specification or written report drawn up by experts based on the consolidated results of scientific study, technology, and experience, aimed at optimum benefits and approved by a recognized and representative body.

STANDARD DEVIATION A measure of dispersion or variation. It is the most widely used measure of dispersion of a frequency distribution. It is equal to the positive square root of the variance. The mean tells where the values for a group are centered. The standard deviation is a summary of how widely dispersed the values are around this center.

STANDARD ERROR The standard deviation of an estimate.

STANDARD POPULATION A population in which the age and sex composition is known precisely, as a result of a census or by an arbitrary means—e.g., an imaginary population, the "standard million," in which age/sex composition is arbitrary. A standard population is used as a comparison group in the actuarial procedure of standardization of mortality rates.

STANDARDIZATION A set of techniques used to remove as far as possible the effects of differences in age or other confounding variables when comparing two or more populations. The common method uses weighted averaging of rates specific for age, sex, or some other potential confounding variable(s) according to some specified distribution of these variables. There are two main methods, as follows:

Direct method: The specific rates in a study population are averaged, using as weights the distribution of a specified standard population. The directly standardized rate represents what the crude rate would have been in the study population if that population had the same distribution as the standard population with respect to the variable(s) for which the adjustment or standardization was carried out.

Indirect method: This is used to compare study populations for which the specific rates are either statistically unstable or unknown. The specific rates in the standard population are averaged, using as weights the distribution of the study population. The ratio of the crude rate for the study population to the weighted average so obtained is the standardized mortality (or morbidity) ratio, or SMR. The indirectly standardized rate itself is the product of the SMR and the crude rate for the standard population.

STANDARDIZED INCIDENCE RATIO The ratio of the incident number of cases of a specified condition in the study population to the incident number that would be expected if the study population had the same incidence rate as a standard or other population for which the incidence rate is known; this ratio is usually expressed as a percentage.

STANDARDIZED MORTALITY RATIO (SMR) The ratio of the number of deaths observed in the study group or population to the number that would be expected if the study population had the same specific rates as the standard population, multiplied by 100.

STANDARDIZED RATE RATIO (SRR) A rate ratio in which the numerator and denominator rates have been standardized to the same (standard) population distribution.

STANDARD METROPOLITAN STATISTICAL AREA Because of the extensive interactions between a city and its surrounding areas, a unit encompassing both is needed as a base for statistical description. The concept of a standard metropolitan statistical area (SMSA) was introduced in the United States to furnish such a unit. To qualify as an SMSA an area has to meet criteria related to size, social and economic integration of the city and surrounding county or counties, minimum population density, and minimum proportion of the labor force engaged in nonagricultural work.

STATIONARY POPULATION A stable population that has a zero growth rate with constant numbers of births and deaths each year.

STATISTICS The science and art of collecting, summarizing, and analyzing data that are subject to random variation. The term is also applied to the data themselves and to summarizations of the data. Statistical terms are defined by Kendall and Buckland.[1]

[1] Kendall MG, Buckland WR. *A Dictionary of Statistical Terms,* 4th ed. London: Longman, 1982.

STATISTICAL ERROR See ERROR.

STATISTICAL INFERENCE See INFERENCE.

STATISTICAL MODEL See MATHEMATICAL MODEL.

STATISTICAL SIGNIFICANCE Statistical methods allow an estimate to be made of the probability of the observed or greater degree of association between independent and dependent variables under the null hypothesis. From this estimate, in a sample of given size, the statistical "significance" of a result can be stated. Usually the level of statistical significance is stated by the P VALUE.

STATISTICAL TEST A procedure that is intended to decide whether a hypothesis about the distribution of one or more populations or variables should be rejected or accepted. Statistical tests may be parametric or nonparametric.

STEM-AND-LEAF DISPLAY A method, developed by J. Tukey, to present numbers in a form resembling a histogram, with multiples of 10 along the "stem" and the integers forming the "leaves." (See art next page.)

STEREOGRAM (Syn: isometric chart) A graph or chart that displays more than two variables in a manner that appears three-dimensional to the eye.

STOCHASTIC PROCESS A process that incorporates some element of randomness.

STOPPING RULES In randomized controlled trials and other forms of systematic experiments, stopping rules are laid down in advance, specifying conditions or criteria under which the trial or experiment shall cease or be terminated. For example, in a RANDOMIZED CONTROLLED TRIAL, the unequivocal demonstration of superiority of one regimen over another is the most obvious reason for terminating the trial; a less frequent situation is the demonstration that a regimen causes harm to participants in the trial. The rule must be based on appropriate statistical tests to ensure that the empirically observed results are not due to chance.

STRATEGY (1) In game theory, a mathematical function. (2) A set of essential measures (preventive, therapeutic) believed sufficient to control a health problem.

STRATIFICATION The process of or result of separating a sample into several subsamples according to specified criteria such as age groups, socioeconomic status, etc. The effect of confounding variables may be controlled by stratifying the analysis of results. For example, lung cancer is known to be associated with smoking. To examine the possible association between urban atmospheric pollution and lung cancer, controlling for smoking, the population may be divided into strata according to smoking status. The association between air pollution and cancer can then be appraised separately within each stratum. Stratification is used not only to control for confounding effects but also as a way of detecting modifying effects. In this example, stratification makes it possible to examine the effect of smoking on the association between atmospheric pollution and lung cancer.

1987: 226, 307, 350, 236, 222, 258, 197, 167, 138, 108, 191, 190, 201

1988: 216, 238, 331, 270, 265, 156, 164, 142, 112, 111, 153, 138, 159

1989: 145, 306, 314, 264, 222, 195, 155, 149, 102, 117, 174, 158, 159

Stem	Leaf
34	0
32	1
30	674
28	
26	450
24	8
22	22668
20	16
18	0157
16	474
14	259356899
12	88
10	28127

In this example the first two digits of each datum serve as the stem and the third digit serves as a leaf, e.g., for the numbers 264 and 265, the stem and leaves appear as 26 (stem) and 45 (leaves). Since further division of the stems would result in an attenuated distributional shape, each stem represents a range of 20 numbers, e.g., the stem 26 represents any number from 260 to 279 so that for the number 270, the stem and leaf appear as 26 (stem) and 0 (leaf).

Stem and leaf display of 4-week totals of meningococcal infections, United States, 1987–1989. From Teutsch and Churchill, op. cit. With permission.

STRATIFIED RANDOMIZATION (Syn: blocked randomization) A randomization procedure in which strata are identified and subjects randomly allocated within each. This produces a situation intermediate between paired allocation and simple random allocation.

STRUCTURED ABSTRACT A summary description of a study. The structured abstract is intended to provide a logical order for the presentation of a scientific communication. A typical sequence is "Objectives, Design, Setting, Subjects, Main Outcome Measures, Results, Conclusions." Structured abstracts have been adopted by some journals, but not by most journals of epidemiology. See Ad hoc Working Group for Critical Appraisal of the Medical Literature. *Ann Intern Med* 1987; 106:598–604.

STUDY BASE The persons (or person-time) in which the outcome of interest is observed. In case control studies, cases and controls should be representative of the same base experience. Miettinen[1] distinguishes between primary and secondary bases; in the former, the population experience is defined in time and place; in the latter, the cases are defined before the study base is or can be defined.

[1] Miettinen OS. *Theoretical Epidemiology.* New York: Wiley, 1985.

STUDY DESIGN See RESEARCH DESIGN.

SUBCLINICAL DISEASE See DISEASE, SUBCLINICAL.

SUMMATIVE RATING Rating scale based on measurements of individually scaled items that are monotonically related to an underlying attribute or attributes; the sum of the item scores is approximately linearly related to the attribute.

SUPERINFECTION Fresh infection in a host already infected with a parasite of the same species; a term mainly used in malaria epidemiology.

SURVEILLANCE Continuous analysis, interpretation, and feedback of systematically collected data, generally using methods distinguished by their practicality, uniformity, and rapidity rather than by accuracy or completeness.[1] By observing trends in time, place, and persons, changes can be observed or anticipated and appropriate action, including investigative or control measures, can be taken. Sources of data may relate directly to disease or to factors influencing disease. Thus they may include (1) mortality and morbidity reports based on death certificates, hospital records, general practice sentinels, or notifications; (2) laboratory diagnoses; (3) outbreak reports; (4) vaccine utilization–uptake and side effects; (5) sickness absence records; (6) disease determinants such as biological changes in agent, vectors, or reservoirs; (7) susceptibility to disease, as by skin testing or serological surveillance (e.g., serum banks).

[1] Eylenbosch WJ, Noah ND, eds. *Surveillance in Health and Disease.* Oxford, England: Oxford University Press, 1988.

SURVEILLANCE OF DISEASE The continuing scrutiny of all aspects of occurrence and spread of a disease that are pertinent to effective control.

Included are the systematic collection and evaluation of (1) morbidity and mortality reports; (2) special reports of field investigations of epidemics and of individual cases; (3) isolation and identification of infectious agents by laboratories; (4) data concerning the availability, use, and untoward effects of vaccines and toxoids, immune globulins, insecticides, and other substances used in control; (5) information regarding immunity levels in segments of the population; and (6) other relevant epidemiologic data. A report summarizing these data should be prepared and distributed to all cooperating persons and others with a need to know the results of the surveillance activities. The procedure applies to all jurisdictional levels of public health from local to international.[1] Serological surveillance identifies patterns of current and past infection using serological test. See also SEROEPIDEMIOLOGY.

[1] Benenson AS, ed. *Control of Communicable Diseases in Man,* 15th ed. Washington DC: American Public Health Association, 1990.

SURVEY An investigation in which information is systematically collected but in which the experimental method is not used. A population survey may be conducted by face-to-face inquiry, by self-completed questionnaires, by telephone, postal service, or in some other way. Each method has its advantages and disadvantages. For instance, a face-to-face (interview) survey may be a better way than self-completed questionnaire to collect information on attitudes or feelings, but it is more costly. Existing medical or other records may contain accurate information, but not about a representative sample of the population.

The information that is gathered in a survey is usually complex enough to require editing (for accuracy, completeness, etc.), coding, keypunching, i.e., entry on punch cards and processing and analysis nearly always now by computer. The generalizability of results depends upon the extent to which the surveyed population is representative. The term *survey* is sometimes used in a narrow sense to refer specifically to a FIELD SURVEY.

SURVEY INSTRUMENT The interview schedule, questionnaire, medical examination record form, etc., used in a survey.

SURVIVAL ANALYSIS A class of statistical procedures for estimating the SURVIVAL FUNCTION, and for making inferences about the effects on it of treatments, prognostic factors, exposures, and other covariates.

SURVIVAL CURVE A curve that starts at 100% of the study population and shows the percentage of the population still surviving at successive times for as long as information is available. May be applied not only to survival as such, but also to the persistence of freedom from a disease, or complication or some other endpoint.

SURVIVAL FUNCTION (Syn: survival distribution) A function of time, usually denoted by $S(t)$, that starts with a population 100% well at a particular time and provides the percentage of the population still well at later times. Survival functions may be applied to any discrete event, for example, disease incidence or relapse, death, or recovery after onset of disease (in which case the population is initially 100% diseased, and the "survival" function gives the percentage still diseased).

SURVIVAL RATE (Syn: cumulative survival rate) The proportion of survivors in a group, e.g., of patients, studied and followed over a period. The proportion of persons in a specified group alive at the beginning of the time interval (e.g., a 5-year period) who survive to the end of the interval. It is equal to 1 minus the CUMULATIVE DEATH RATE. May be studied by current or cohort LIFE TABLE methods.

SURVIVAL RATIO The probability of surviving between one age and another; when computed for age groups, the ratios correspond to those of the person-years-lived function of a life table.

SURVIVORSHIP STUDY Use of a cohort LIFE TABLE to provide the probability that an event, such as death, will occur in successive intervals of time after diagnosis and, conversely, the probability of surviving each interval. The multiplication of these probabilities of survival for each time interval for those alive at the beginning of that interval yields a cumulative probability of surviving for the total period of study.

SUSCEPTIBLE VARIABLE A variable that is potentially confounding in that it is subsequent, not antecedent, to the variable whose effect is being studied. A susceptible variable may or may not be an intervening variable.

SYMBIOSIS The biological association of two or more species to their mutual benefit.

SYMMETRICAL RELATIONSHIP An association between variables that does not have direction.

The following varieties can be distinguished:
1. Functional interdependence, where one variable cannot exist without the other; e.g., prevalence is a function of incidence and duration.
2. Common complex, where variables occur together without being interdependent or necessary to each other; e.g., the occurrence together of air pollution, poverty, poor housing, and overcrowding.
3. Alternative indicators of the same entity; e.g., antibodies to a microorganism and history of specific infection caused by that microorganism.
4. The effects of a common cause; e.g., clinical and biochemical changes in hepatitis.

See also ASSOCIATION, SYMMETRICAL.

SYNDROME A symptom complex in which the symptoms and/or signs coexist more frequently than would be expected by chance on the assumption of independence.

SYNERGISM, SYNERGY
1. A situation in which the combined effect of two or more factors is greater than the sum of their solitary effects.
2. In BIOASSAY, two factors act synergistically if there are persons who will get the disease when exposed to both factors but not when exposed to either alone. ANTAGONISM, the opposite of synergism, exists if there are persons who will get the disease when exposed to one of the factors alone, but not when exposed to

both. Note that under these definitions two factors may act synergistically in some persons and antagonistically in others.

SYSTEMATIC ERROR See BIAS.

SYSTEMS ANALYSIS This term is used with three similar meanings:

1. The examination of various elements of a system with a view to ascertaining whether the proposed solution to a problem will fit into the system and, in turn, effect an overall improvement in the system.
2. The analysis of an activity in order to determine precisely what is required of the system, how this can best be accomplished, and in what ways the computer can be useful.
3. *Systems analysis* refers to any formal analysis whose purpose is to suggest a course of action by systematically examining the objectives, costs, effectiveness and risks of alternative policies or strategies and designing additional ones if those examined are found wanting. It is an approach to or way of looking at complex problems of choice under uncertainty; it is not yet a method.

T

TARGET An aspired outcome that is explicitly stated, e.g., what a health promotion program will achieve by a specified date: for example, reduced unwanted pregnancy rates, lower teenage smoking rates, enhanced QALYs. Usually expressed in quantitative terms.

TARGET POPULATION
1. The collection of individuals, items, measurements, etc., about which we want to make inferences. The term is sometimes used to indicate the population from which a sample is drawn and sometimes to denote any "reference" population about which inferences are required.
2. The group of persons for whom an intervention is planned.

TAXON (plural, taxa) The general term for a group or entity, e.g., a species or family in a taxonomy.

TAXONOMY A systematic classification into related groups.

TAXONOMY OF DISEASE The orderly classification of diseases into appropriate categories on the basis of relationships among them, with the application of names. See also NOSOGRAPHY, NOSOLOGY.

t-**DISTRIBUTION,** *t*-**TEST** The *t*-distribution is the distribution of a quotient of independent random variables, the numerator of which is a standardized normal variate and the denominator of which is the positive square root of the quotient of a chi-square distributed variate and its number of degrees of freedom. The *t*-test uses a statistic that, under the null hypothesis, has the *t*-distribution, to test whether two means differ significantly, or to test linear regression or correlation coefficients. The *t*-distribution and the *t*-test were developed by W. S. Gossett, who wrote under the pseudonym "Student," as his employment precluded individual publication.

TELEOLOGY The philosophical belief that everything occurring in nature has a purpose.

TERATOGEN A substance that produces abnormalities in the embryo or fetus by disturbing maternal homeostasis or by acting directly on the fetus in utero.

TEST OF SIGNIFICANCE See P VALUE; STATISTICAL SIGNIFICANCE.

TEST HYPOTHESIS See NULL HYPOTHESIS.

THEORETICAL EPIDEMIOLOGY The development of mathematical/statistical models to explain different aspects of the occurrence of a variety of diseases. With some infectious diseases, models have been generated to elucidate the reasons for epidemics and/or to predict the behavior of the disease in reaction to given control measures. See also MODEL.

THERAPEUTIC TRIAL See CLINICAL TRIAL.

THRESHOLD LIMIT VALUE See SAFETY STANDARDS.

THRESHOLD PHENOMENA Events or changes that occur only after a certain level of a characteristic is reached.

TIME CLUSTER See CLUSTERING.

TIME-PLACE CLUSTER See CLUSTERING.

TOLERANCE In toxicology, the adaptive state characterized by diminished effects of a particular dose of a substance.

TORT A legal term for the harmful consequence of an act. Such acts are tried in courts of law, and damages are awarded if wrong or harm is demonstrated. A "toxic tort" is a lawsuit centered around a claim for harm due to a toxic chemical. Epidemiologists sometimes have to testify in legal cases involving tort.

TOTAL FERTILITY RATE (TFR) The average number of children that would be born per woman if all women lived to the end of their childbearing years and bore children according to a given set of age-specific fertility rates. It is computed by summing the age-specific fertility rates for all ages and multiplying by the interval into which the ages are grouped. The TFR is an important fertility measure, providing the most accurate answer to the question, "How many children does a women have, on average?"

TOWNSEND SCORE An index of social deprivation developed by the British social scientist Peter Townsend (1928–   ), used mainly in the UK; based on numbers economically active but unemployed, households with no car, households not owner-occupied, households overcrowded. The Townsend score uses readily available census data and can be used to rank administratively defined jurisdictions. See also OVERCROWDING.

Townsend P, Phillimore P, Beattie A. *Health and Deprivation: Inequality and the North.* London: Croom Helm, 1988.

TOXICOLOGY The scientific discipline involving the study of actual or potential danger presented by the harmful effects of chemicals (poisons) on living organisms and ecosystems, of the relationship of such harmful effects to exposure, and of the mechanisms of action, diagnosis, prevention, and treatment of intoxications. (From IUPAC Glossary.) Toxicology has an increasingly broad interface with epidemiology.

TRACER DISEASE METHOD Tracer or indicator conditions as defined by Kessner[1] are easily diagnosed, reasonably frequent illnesses or health states whose outcomes are believed to be affected by health care and which taken in aggregate should reflect the gamut of patients and health problems encountered in a medical practice. The extent to which the recorded care of these conditions concurs with preset standards of care is used as an index of the quality of care delivered. However, it should first be shown that the preset standards contribute to a favorable outcome. See also SENTINEL HEALTH EVENT.

[1] Kessner DM, Snow CK, Singer J. *Assessment of Medical Care for Children.* Washington DC: National Academy of Sciences, Institute of Medicine, 1974.

TRANSCRIPTION Copying of a strand of DNA to generate a complementary strand of RNA.

TRANSMISSION OF INFECTION Transmission of infectious agents. Any mechanism by which an infectious agent is spread from a source or reservoir to another person. These mechanisms are defined as follows:

1. Direct transmission

   Direct and essentially immediate transfer of infectious agents to a receptive portal of entry through which human or animal infection may take place. This may be by direct contract as by touching, kissing, biting, or sexual intercourse, or by the direct projection (droplet spread) of droplet spray onto the conjunctiva or onto the mucous membranes of the eyes, nose, or mouth during sneezing, coughing, spitting, singing, or talking (usually limited to a distance of about 1 m or less). It may also be by direct exposure of susceptible tissue to an agent in soil, compost, or decaying vegetable matter in which it normally leads a saprophytic existence, (e.g., the systemic mycoses), or by the bite of a rabid animal. Transplacental transmission is another form of direct transmission.

2. Indirect transmission

Vehicle-borne—Contaminated inanimate material or objects (fomites) such as toys, handkerchiefs, soiled clothes, bedding, cooking or eating utensils, and surgical instruments or dressings (indirect contact); water, food, milk, biological products including blood, serum, plasma, tissues, or organs; or any substance serving as an intermediate means by which an infectious agent is transported and introduced into a susceptible host through a suitable portal of entry. The agent may or may not have multiplied or developed in or on the vehicle before being transmitted.

Vector-borne—(a) *Mechanical:* Includes simple mechanical carriage by a crawling or flying insect through soiling of its feet or proboscis, or by passage of organisms through its gastrointestinal tract. This does not require multiplication or development of the organism. (b) *Biological:* Propagation (multiplication), cyclic development, or a combination of these (cyclopropagative) is required before the arthropod can transmit the infective form of the agent to man. An incubation period (extrinsic) is required following infection before the arthropod becomes infective. The infectious agent may be passed vertically to succeeding generations (transovarian transmission); transstadial transmission is its passage from the one stage of the life cycle to another, as nymph to adult. Transmission may be by saliva during biting or by regurgitation or deposition on the skin of feces or other material capable of penetrating subsequently through the bite wound or through an area of trauma from scratching or rubbing. This is transmission by an infected nonvertebrate host and must be differentiated for epidemiologic purposes from simple mechanical carriage by a vector in the role of a vehicle. An arthropod in either role is termed a *vector.*

Airborne—The dissemination of microbial aerosols to a suitable portal of entry, usually the respiratory tract. Microbial aerosols are suspensions in the air of particles consisting partially or wholly of microorganisms. Particles in the 1 to 5μ range are easily drawn into the alveoli of the lungs and may be retained there; many are exhaled from the alveoli without deposition. They may remain suspended in the air for long periods of time, some retaining and others losing infectivity or virulence. Not considered as airborne are droplets and other large particles that promptly settle out (see *Direct transmission,* above).

The following are airborne and their mode of transmission is direct:

Droplet nuclei: Usually the small residues that result from evaporation of fluid from droplets emitted by an infected host (see above). Droplet nuclei also may be created purposely by a variety of atomizing devices, or accidentally as in microbiology laboratories or in abattoirs, rendering plants, or autopsy rooms. They usually remain suspended in the air for long periods of time.

Dust: The small particles of widely varying size that may arise from soil (as, for example, fungus spores separated from dry soil by wind or mechanical agitation), clothes, bedding, or contaminated floors.[1] See also ACQUAINTANCE NETWORK; AIRBORNE INFECTION; CARRIER; COMMON VEHICLE SPREAD; CONTACT; CONTAMINATION; DROPLET NUCLEI.

[1] Benenson AS, ed. *Control of Communicable Diseases in Man,* 15th ed. Washington DC: American Public Health Association, 1990.

TRANSMISSION PARAMETER *(r)* In infectious disease epidemiology, the proportion of total possible contacts between infectious cases and susceptibles that lead to new infections.

TRANSOVARIAL TRANSMISSION See VECTOR-BORNE INFECTION.

TRANSPORT HOST See PARATENIC HOST.

TREND A long-term movement in an ordered series, e.g., a time series. An essential feature is that the movement, while possibly irregular in the short term, shows movement consistently in the same direction over a long term. The term is also used loosely to refer to an association which is consistent in several samples or strata but is not statistically significant.

TREND LINE The line that best fits the distribution of a set of values plotted on two axes.

TRIAGE The process of selecting for care or treatment those of highest priority or, when resources are limited, those thought most likely to benefit. From the French, *trier*, to separate, choose.

TRIAL See CLINICAL TRIAL.

"TRIMMING" (data trimming) The practice, which can be akin to a form of scientific fraud or misrepresentation, of excluding from analysis observations or measurements that lie outside the range the investigator expects; the grounds for exclusion are that these outlying observations would distort the results. Data trimming is permissible only when rules written in advance in the research protocol specify circumstances in which it may be done. Even then it should be done with caution, and openly. See also OUTLIERS.

TRIPLE BLIND A study in which the subjects, observers, and analysts are blinded as to which subjects received what interventions.

TROHOC STUDY A retrospective case control study. The term, proposed by A. R. Feinstein,[1] is the inversion of "cohort;" its use is deprecated by the great majority of epidemiologists.

[1] *Clin Pharmacol Ther* 1981; 30:564–577.

TUBERCULOSIS A chronic disease since Neolithic times, afflicting an estimated 1.7 billion people, one-third of the world's population, caused by *Mycobacterium tuberculosis*. It merits mention in this dictionary because it presents an increasing epidemiologic challenge[1]—the tuberculin skin test, which has long been a simple, cheap means of screening, is less efficient in populations that have been vaccinated with BCG and in which there are large numbers of immunocompromised persons infected with HIV.

[1] Porter JDH, McAdam KPWJ. The re-emergence of tuberculosis. *Annu Rev Public Health* 1994; 15:303–323.

TUKEY'S METHOD See MULTIPLE COMPARISON TECHNIQUES.

TWIN STUDY Method of detecting genetic etiology in human disease. The basic premise of twin studies is that monozygotic twins, being formed by the division of a single fertilized ovum, carry identical genes, while dizygotic twins, being formed by the fertilization of two ova by two different spermatozoa, are genetically no more similar than two siblings born after separate pregnancies.

TWO-TAIL TEST A statistical significance test based on the assumption that the data are distributed in both directions from some central value(s).

TYPE I ERROR See ERROR.

TYPE II ERROR See ERROR.

"TYPHOID MARY" A jargon term for an individual who unwittingly transmits infection to others. The original Typhoid Mary, Mary Mallon, was an itinerant cook and an infamous carrier of typhoid in New York City and environs early in the 20th century.

U, V

UNBIASED ESTIMATOR An estimator that for all sample sizes has an expected value equal to the parameter being estimated. If an estimator tends to be unbiased as sample size increases, it is referred to as asymptotically unbiased.

UNDERLYING CAUSE OF DEATH The disease or injury that initiated the train of events leading directly to death, or the circumstances of the accident or violence that produced the fatal injury. See DEATH CERTIFICATE.

UNDERREPORTING Failure to identify and/or count all cases, leading to reduction of numerator in a rate. See also ERROR.

UNIVERSAL PRECAUTIONS Procedures to be followed when health workers anticipate the possibility of infection by a patient who may harbor a highly contagious, dangerous pathogen. Universal precautions may include segregation of the patient in a private room; use of gloves, gown, mask, Perspex shield (eye protection); and rigorous attention to ensuring that no blood or other body fluid from such a patient can come into contact with skin or mucous membranes of the health care worker. See also NEEDLESTICK.

UNIVERSE See POPULATION.

UNOBTRUSIVE MEASURES A set of methods for assessing behavior without actually asking people how they behave or examining them physically to determine the effects of their behavior.[1] For example, the cigarette smoking behavior of groups can be assessed by studying cigarette sales or by measuring the length of cigarette butts in ashtrays.

[1] Webb EJ, Campbell DT, Schwartz RD, Sechrest L. *Unobtrusive Measures.* Chicago: Rand McNally, 1966.

UTILITY In economics, this term means preference for or desirability of a particular outcome. In decision theory and clinical decision analysis, the term refers to being or becoming healthy rather than sick or disabled. Utility is measured by various means, e.g., QALYs.

UTILITY-BASED UNITS In the context of QUALITY-ADJUSTED LIFE YEARS, utility-based units relate to a person's level of well-being, estimated on the basis of the total life years gained from a procedure or intervention.

VACCINATION Strictly speaking, vaccination refers to inoculation (from Latin *in oculus,* into a bud) with vaccinia virus against smallpox. Nowadays the word is broadly used synonymously with procedures for immunization against all infectious disease. The original use of the word was confined to vaccination against smallpox. This was the first method of preventing a lethal disease by immunizing humans. It was introduced by Edward Jenner (1749–1823) and described by him in *An Inquiry into the Cause and Effects of the Variolae Vaccinae* (1798). Jenner's discovery led directly to the worldwide eradication of smallpox.

VACCINE Immunobiological substance used for active immunization by introducing into

170

the body a live modified, attenuated, or killed inactivated infectious organism or its toxin. The vaccine is capable of stimulating immune response by the host, who is thus rendered resistant to infection. The word *vaccine* was originally applied to the serum from a cow infected with vaccinia virus (cowpox; from Latin *vacca,* cow); it is now used of all immunizing agents.

VACCINE EFFICACY (Syn: protective efficacy). Mathematically, this is defined as the proportion of persons in the placebo group of a vaccine trial who would not have become ill if they had received the vaccine; alternatively it is the percentage reduction of cases among vaccinated individuals.

VALIDATION The process of establishing that a method is sound.

VALIDITY This term, derived from the Latin *validus,* strong, has several meanings usually accompanied by a qualifying word or phrase.

VALIDITY, MEASUREMENT An expression of the degree to which a measurement measures what it purports to measure.

Several varieties are distinguished, including construct validity, content validity, and criterion validity (concurrent and predictive validity).

Construct validity: The extent to which the measurement corresponds to theoretical concepts (constructs) concerning the phenomenon under study. For example, if on theoretical grounds, the phenomenon should change with age, a measurement with construct validity would reflect such a change.

Content validity: The extent to which the measurement incorporates the domain of the phenomenon under study. For example, a measurement of functional health status should embrace activities of daily living, occupational, family, and social functioning, etc.

Criterion validity: The extent to which the measurement correlates with an external criterion of the phenomenon under study. Two aspects of criterion validity can be distinguished:

1. *Concurrent validity:* The measurement and the criterion refer to the same point in time. An example is a visual inspection of a wound for evidence of infection validated against bacteriological examination of a specimen taken at the same time.
2. *Predictive validity:* The measurement's validity is expressed in terms of its ability to predict the criterion. An example is an academic aptitude test that is validated against subsequent academic performance.

VALIDITY, STUDY The degree to which the inference drawn from a study, especially generalizations extending beyond the study sample, are warranted when account is taken of the study methods, the representativeness of the study sample, and the nature of the population from which it is drawn. Two varieties of study validity are distinguished:

1. *Internal validity:* The index and comparison groups are selected and compared in such a manner that the observed differences between them on the dependent variables under study may, apart from sampling error, be attributed only to the hypothesized effect under investigation.
2. *External validity (generalizability):* A study is externally valid or generalizable if it can produce unbiased inferences regarding a target population (beyond the subjects in the study). This aspect of validity is only meaningful with regard to a specified external target population. For example, the results of a study conducted using only white male subjects might or might not be generalizable to all human males (the target population consisting of all human males). It is not generalizable to females (the target population consisting of all people).

The evaluation of generalizability usually involves much more subject-matter judgment than internal validity.

These epidemiologic definitions of the terms *internal validity* and *external validity* do not correspond exactly to some definitions found in the sociological literature. See also CRITICAL APPRAISAL, EVIDENCE-BASED MEDICINE.

VALUES

1. In sociology, what we believe in, what we hold dear about the way we live. Our values influence our behavior as persons, groups, communities, cultures—perhaps as a species. Values therefore are an important determinant of individual and community health; they are, however, difficult to measure objectively except unobtrusively.
2. In statistics, magnitude of measurements.

VARIABLE Any quantity that varies. Any attribute, phenomenon, or event that can have different values.

VARIABLE, ANTECEDENT A variable that causally precedes the association or outcome under study. See also EXPLANATORY VARIABLE; INDEPENDENT VARIABLE.

VARIABLE, CONFOUNDING See CONFOUNDING.

VARIABLE, CONTROL Independent variable other than the "hypothetical causal variable" that has a potential effect on the dependent variable and is subject to control by analysis.

VARIABLE, DEPENDENT See DEPENDENT VARIABLE.

VARIABLE, DISTORTER A CONFOUNDING VARIABLE that diminishes, masks, or reverses the association under study.

VARIABLE, EXPERIENTIAL See INDEPENDENT VARIABLE.

VARIABLE INDEPENDENT See INDEPENDENT VARIABLE.

VARIABLE, INTERVENING See INTERVENING VARIABLE.

VARIABLE, MANIFESTATIONAL See DEPENDENT VARIABLE.

VARIABLE, MODERATOR See EFFECT MODIFIER.

VARIABLE, PASSENGER See PASSENGER VARIABLE.

VARIABLE, UNCONTROLLED A (potentially) confounding variable that has not been brought under control by design or analysis. See also CONFOUNDING.

VARIANCE A measure of the variation shown by a set of observations, defined by the sum of the squares of deviation from the mean, divided by the number of DEGREES OF FREEDOM in the set of observations.

VARIATE (Syn: random variable) A variable that may assume any of a set of values, each with a preassigned probability (known as its distribution).

VECTOR

1. In infectious disease epidemiology, an insect or any living carrier that transports an infectious agent from an infected individual or its wastes to a susceptible individual or its food or immediate surroundings. The organism may or may not pass through a developmental cycle within the vector.
2. In statistics, an ordered set of numbers representing the values of a set of variables.

VECTOR-BORNE INFECTION Several classes of vector-borne infections are recognized, each with epidemiologic features that are determined by the interaction between the infectious agent and the human host, on the one hand, and the vector on the other. Therefore, environmental factors such as climatic and seasonal variations influence the epidemiologic pattern by virtue of their effects on the vector and its habits.

The terms used to describe specific features of vector-borne infections are:

Biological transmission: Transmission of the infectious agent to susceptible host by bite of blood-feeding (arthropod) vector as in malaria, or by other inoculation, as in *Schistosoma* infection.

Extrinsic incubation period: Time necessary after acquisition of infection by the (arthropod) vector for the infectious agent to multiply or develop sufficiently so that it can be transmitted by the vector to a vertebrate host.

Hibernation: A possible mechanism by which the infected vector survives adverse cold weather by becoming dormant.

Inapparent infection: Response to infection without developing overt signs of illness. If this is accompanied by viremia or bacteremia in a high proportion of infected animals or persons, the receptor species is well suited as an epidemiologically important host in the transmission cycle.

Mechanical transmission: Transport of the infectious agent between hosts by arthropod vectors with contaminated mouthparts, antennae, or limbs. There is no multiplication of the infectious agent in the vector.

Overwintering: Persistence of the infectious microorganism in the vector for extended periods, such as the cooler winter months, during which the vector has no opportunity to be reinfected or to infect a vertebrate host. Overwintering is an important concept in the epidemiology of vector-borne diseases since the annual recrudescence of viral activity after periods (winter, dry season) adverse to continual transmission depends upon a mechanism for local survival of an infectious microorganism or its reintroduction from outside the endemic area. To some extent, the risk of a summertime epidemic may be determined by the relative success of microorganism survival in the local winter reservoir. Since overwinter survival may in turn depend upon the level of activity of the microorganism during the preceding summer and autumn, outbreaks sometimes occur for two or more successive years.

Transovarial infection (transmission): Transmission of the infectious microorganism from the affected female arthropod to her progeny.

VECTOR SPACE An area (or volume) defined by the specified dimensions of two (or three) vectors.

VEHICLE OF INFECTION TRANSMISSION The mode of transmission of an infectious agent from its reservoir to a susceptible host. This can be person-to-person, food, vector-borne, etc.

VENN DIAGRAM A pictorial presentation of the extent to which two or more quantities or concepts are mutually inclusive and exclusive.

VERBAL AUTOPSY A procedure for gathering systematic information that enables a determination to be made of the cause of death in situations where the deceased has not been medically attended. It is based on the assumption that most common and important causes of death have distinct symptom complexes that can be recognized, remembered, and reported by lay respondents. It is a useful way to enhance the quality of mortality statistics in developing countries.[1]

[1] Chandramohan D, Maude GH, Rodriques LC, Hayes RJ. Verbal autopsies for adult deaths: Issues in their development and validation. *Int J Epidemiol* 1994; 23:213–230.

VIOLENCE Harm caused by the use of force. The harm takes the form of traumatic injury or death. Epidemiologically two main varieties, unintentional and intentional violence, can be distinguished; the former occurs mainly in traffic and industry, the latter mainly in warfare and in domestic settings.

VIRGIN POPULATION A population that has never been exposed to a particular infectious agent.

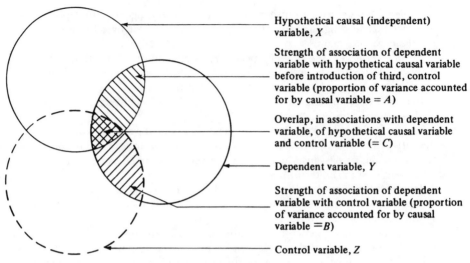

Hypothetical causal (independent) variable, X

Strength of association of dependent variable with hypothetical causal variable before introduction of third, control variable (proportion of variance accounted for by causal variable $= A$)

Overlap, in associations with dependent variable, of hypothetical causal variable and control variable ($= C$)

Dependent variable, Y

Strength of association of dependent variable with control variable (proportion of variance accounted for by causal variable $= B$)

Control variable, Z

Venn diagram.

VIRULENCE The degree of pathogenicity; the disease-evoking power of a microorganism in a given host. Numerically expressed as the ratio of the number of cases of overt infection to the total number infected, as determined by immunoassay. When death is the only criterion of severity, this is the case-fatality rate.

VITAL RECORDS (Literally, "To do with living") Certificates of birth, death, marriage, and divorce required for legal and demographic purposes.

VITAL STATISTICS Systematically tabulated information concerning births, marriages, divorces, separations, and deaths based on registrations of these vital events.

W, X, Y, Z

WASHOUT PHASE That stage in a study, especially a therapeutic trial, when treatment is withdrawn so that its effects disappear and the subject's characteristics return to their baseline state.

WESTERN BLOT See BLOT.

WEIBULL MODEL Dose-response model of the form

$$P(d) = 1 - \exp(-bd^m)$$

where $P(d)$ is the probability of response due to a continuous dose rate d; b and m are constants. The model is useful for extrapolating from high- to low-dose exposures—e.g., animal to human, or occupational to environmental.

WEIGHTED AVERAGE A value determined by assigning weights to individual measurements. Each value is assigned a nonnegative coefficient (weight); the sum of the products of each value by its weight divided by the sum of the weights is the weighted average.

"WHISTLE-BLOWING" Informing authorities or the media when fraud or misrepresentation of research results or any other form of wrongdoing is suspected. The lot of the whistle blower is often unhappy: many have been victimized by the authorities to whom they complain, while the miscreant goes free.

WORKUP BIAS Bias due to incorrectly or incompletely diagnosed cases being more numerous in one group than another in a study in which comparison is made between groups. Usually this happens because patients with a positive screening-level test receive a more thorough workup with diagnostic ("GOLD STANDARD") tests than those whose screening-level test was negative.[1]

[1] Ransohoff DF, Feinstein AR. Problems of spectrum and bias in evaluating the efficacy of diagnostic tests. *N Engl J Med* 1978; 199: 926–930.

WORM COUNT A method of surveillance of helminth infection of the gut that depends upon counts of worms, or their cysts or ova, in quantitatively titrated samples of feces. Other terms used to describe this form of surveillance are *egg count, cyst count,* and *parasite count.*

XENOBIOTIC
1. (Syn: commensal, symbiosis) Pertaining to association of two animal species, usually insects, in the absence of a dependency relationship, as opposed to parasitism.
2. A foreign compound that is metabolized in the body. Many pesticides and their derivatives, some food additives, and a number of other complex organic compounds such as dioxins and PCBs are xenobiotics.

XENODIAGNOSIS Detection of a (human) pathogenic organism by allowing a noninfected vector (e.g., mosquito) to consume infected material, and then examining this vector for evidence of the pathogen.

X-LINKED (Syn: sex-linked) Heritable characteristic transmitted by a gene located on the X chromosome.

YATES' CORRECTION An adjustment proposed by Yates (1934) in the chi-square calculation for a 2×2 table, which brings the distribution based on discontinuous frequencies closer to the continuous chi-square distribution from which the published tables for testing chi-squares are derived

YEARS OF POTENTIAL LIFE LOST (YPLL) See POTENTIAL YEARS OF LIFE LOST.

YIELD The number or proportion of cases of a condition accurately identified by a screening test.

YOUDEN'S INDEX When assessing screening tests, in the uncommon case where the risk of a false negative and that of a false positive result are assumed to be equivalent (i.e., specificity and sensitivity assumed to be equally important), it may be possible to compare screening tests through the Youden index based on the sum of specificity and sensitivity:

$$\text{Youden index} = J = \text{specificity} + \text{sensitivity} - 1$$

with J ranging from zero (specificity = 0.50 and sensitivity = 0.50) to 1 (sensitivity = 1.00, specificity = 1.00).

ZELEN DESIGN (Syn: prerandomization design) A modified double-blind RANDOMIZED CONTROLLED TRIAL design proposed by Marvin Zelen (1927–). The essential feature of the Zelen design is randomization before informed consent procedures, which are claimed to be needed only for the group allocated to receive the experimental regimen. Many ethicists disagree, holding that it is necessary to obtain the informed consent of all participants, regardless of the group to which they are allocated.

ZERO POPULATION GROWTH The status of a population in which there is no net increase of numbers; the number of births (plus immigrants) equals the number of deaths (plus emigrants).

ZERO SUM GAME A situation in which one participant can "gain" only at the expense of or to the detriment of another.

ZERO-TIME SHIFT This concerns the selection of a starting point for the measurement of survival following the detection of disease. It is a jargon term, denoting the movement "backward" (toward the starting point of a disease) of time between onset and detection, that may accompany use of a screening procedure.

ZOONOSIS An infection or infectious disease transmissible under natural conditions from vertebrate animals to humans. Examples include rabies and plague. May be enzootic or epizootic.

Z SCORE Score expressed as a deviation from the mean value, in standard deviation units; the term is used in analyzing continuous variables such as heights and weights of a sample, to express results of behavioral tests, etc.

Bibliography

Dictionaries, glossaries, general reference works

The Compact Oxford English Dictionary (OED), new ed. Oxford and New York: Oxford University Press, 1991.

Webster's Third New International Dictionary. Springfield, MA: Merriam, 1971.

Allaby M. *Dictionary of the Environment.* Southampton, England: London Press, 1975.

Bander EJ, Wallach JJ. *Medical Legal Dictionary.* Dobbs Ferry, NY: Oceana, 1970.

Campbell RJ, ed. *Psychiatric Dictionary,* 5th ed. New York: Oxford University Press, 1981.

Duffus JH, ed, for the International Union of Pure and Applied Chemistry. *Glossary for Chemists of Terms Used in Toxicology* (IUPAC Recommendations, 1993). Published in *Pure Appl Chem* 1993; 65:2003–2122.

Feinstein AR. A Glossary of neologisms in quantitative clinical science. *Clin Pharmacol Ther* 1981; 30:564–577.

Froom J. An international glossary for primary care. *J Fam Pract* 1981; 13:673–681.

Glossary of Health Services; Terminology Bulletin No. 205. Ottawa: Secretary of State, 1991.

Goldstein AS. *Dictionary of Health Care Administration.* Rockville, MD: Aspen, 1989.

Hogarth J. *Glossary of Health Care Terminology.* Copenhagen: World Health Organization, 1975.

Holland WW, Detels R, Knox G, eds. *The Oxford Testbook of Public Health,* 2nd ed. Oxford and New York: Oxford University Press, 1991.

Jammal A, Allard R, Loslier G, eds. *Dictionnaire d'épidémiologie.* Ste-Hyacinthe, Maloine, Paris: Edisem, 1988.

Kendall MG, Buckland WR. *A Dictionary of Statistical Terms,* 4th ed. London and New York: Longman, 1982.

King RC, Stansfield WD. *A Dictionary of Genetics,* 4th ed. New York: Oxford University Press, 1990.

Landau SI, ed. *International Dictionary of Medicine and Biology.* New York: Wiley, 1986.

Last JM, Wallace RB, eds. *Maxcy-Rosenau-Last Public Health and Preventive Medicine,* 13th ed. Norwalk, CT: Appleton & Lange, 1992.

Leclerk A, Papoz L, Bréart G, Lellouch J. *Dictionnaire d'épidémiologie.* Paris: Frison-Roche, 1990.

Meadows AJ, Gordon M, Singleton A. *A Dictionary of New Information Technology.* London: Century, 1982.

Morton LG, ed. *Garrison & Morton's Medical Bibliography,* 4th ed. London: Gower, 1983.

Pressat R. *Dictionnaire de Démographie* (The Dictionary of Demography). English translation edited by Christopher Wilson. Oxford: Blackwell, 1985.

Segen JC, ed. *Dictionary of Modern Medicine*. Camforth, UK, and Park Ridge NJ: Parthenon, 1992.

Skinner HA. *The Origin of Medical Terms,* 2nd ed. Baltimore, MD: Williams & Wilkins 1961.

Sohm ED, ed. *Glossary of Evaluation Terms*. Geneva: United Nations, 1978.

Stedman's Medical Dictionary, 25th ed. Baltimore, MD: Williams & Wilkins, 1990.

Thériault Y, Beauregard E, Charuest M. *Statistics and Surveys Vocabulary;* Terminology Bulletin No. 208. Ottawa: Secretary of State, 1992.

Toma B, Bénet JJ, Dufour B, Eloit M, et al. *Glossaire d'épidémiologie animale*. Maisons-Alfort, France: Editions du Point Vétérinaire, 1991.

US House of Representatives, 94th Congress, *A Discursive Dictionary of Health Care*. Washington, DC: USGPO, 1976.

Vogt WP. *Dictionary of Statistics and Methodology*. Newbury Park, London: Sage 1993.

van de Walle E. *Multilingual Demographic Dictionary,* English section, 2nd ed. Liège, Belgium: Ordina, 1982.

Wolman BB, ed. *Dictionary of Behavioral Science*. New York: Van Nostrand, 1973.

World Bank. *A Glossary of Population Terminology*. Washington, DC: World Bank, 1985.

Monographs and collections on epidemiology, biostatistics, etc.

Abramson JH, *Survey Methods in Community Medicine,* 4th ed. London: Churchill Livingstone, 1990.

Abramson JH, *Making Sense of Data,* 2nd ed. New York: Oxford University Press, 1994.

Armstrong BK, White E, Saracci R. *Principles of Exposure Measurement in Epidemiology*. Oxford, New York, Melbourne: Oxford Medical Publications, 1992.

Bailar III JC, Mosteller F. *Medical Uses of Statistics*. Boston: New England Journal of Medicine Books, 1986.

Barker DJP, Rose G. *Epidemiology in Medical Practice,* 3rd ed. Edinburgh: Churchill Livingstone, 1992.

Beaglehole R, Bonita R, Kjellström T. *Basic Epidemiology*. Geneva: World Health Organization, 1993.

Benenson AS, ed. *Control of Communicable Diseases in Man,* 15th ed. Washington, DC: American Public Health Association, 1990.

Bernier RH, Mason VM. *Episource: a Guide to Resources in Epidemiology*. Roswell, GA: Epidemiology Monitor, 1991.

Breslow NE, Day NE. *Statistical Methods in Cancer Research:* Vol 1. *The Analysis of Case-Control Data*. Lyon: IARC, 1980. Vol. 2. *The Design and Analysis of Cohort Studies*. Lyon: IARC, 1987.

Committee on Environmental Epidemiology, Commission on Life Sciences, National Research Council. *Environmental Epidemiology*. Washington, DC: National Academy Press, Vol 1, 1991; Vol 2, 1995

Dawson-Saunders B, Trapp RG. *Basic and Clinical Biostatistics,* 2nd ed. Norwalk, CT: Appleton & Lange, 1994.

Elliott P, Cuzick J, English D, Stern R. *Geographical and Environmental Epidemiology: Methods for Small-Area Studies*. New York: Oxford University Press, 1993.

Elwood JM. *Causal Relationships in Medicine: A Practical System for Critical Appraisal*. Oxford, New York, Melbourne: Oxford Medical Publications, 1988.

Feinstein AR. *Clinical Epidemiology*. Philadelphia: Saunders, 1985.

Fleiss JL. *Statistical Methods for Rates and Proportions,* 2nd ed. New York: Wiley, 1981.

Fletcher RH, Fletcher SW, Wagner EH. *Clinical Epidemiology—The Essentials,* 2nd ed. Baltimore, MD: Williams & Wilkins, 1990.

Friedman GD. *Primer of Epidemiology,* 3rd ed. New York: McGraw-Hill, 1987.

Gordis L, ed. *Epidemiology and Health Risk Assessment.* New York: Oxford University Press, 1988.

Greenberg RS, Daniels SR, Flanders WD, et al. *Medical Epidemiology.* Norwalk, CT: Appleton & Lange, 1993.

Hennekens CH, Buring JE, Mayrent SL. *Epidemiology in Medicine.* Boston: Little, Brown, 1987.

Kelsey JL, Thompson WD, Evans AS. *Methods in Observational Epidemiology.* New York: Oxford University Press, 1986.

Kahn HA, Sempos CT. *Statistical Methods in Epidemiology.* New York: Oxford University Press, 1989.

Khoury MJ, Beaty TH, Cohen BH. *Fundamentals of Genetic Epidemiology.* New York: Oxford University Press, 1993.

Kleinbaum DG, Kupper LL, Morgenstern H. *Epidemiology—Principles and Quantitative Methods.* Belmont, CA: Lifetime Learning, 1982.

Last JM. *Public Health and Human Ecology.* Norwalk, CT: Appleton & Lange, 1987.

Lilienfeld DE, Stolley PD. *Foundations of Epidemiology,* 3rd ed. New York: Oxford University Press, 1994.

Meinert CL. *Clinical Trials: Design, Conduct and Analysis.* New York: Oxford University Press, 1986.

Miettinen OS. *Theoretical Epidemiology: Principles of Occurrence Research in Medicine.* New York: Wiley, 1985.

Macmahon B, Pugh TF. *Epidemiology: Principles and Methods.* Boston: Little, Brown, 1970.

McDowell IW, Newell C. *Measuring Health: A Guide to Rating Scales and Questionnaires.* New York: Oxford University Press, 1987.

Monson RR. *Occupational Epidemiology,* 2nd ed. Boca Raton, FL: CRC Press, 1990.

Morrison AS. *Screening in Chronic Disease,* 2nd ed. New York: Oxford University Press, 1992.

Murphy EA. *A Companion to Medical Statistics.* Baltimore, MD: Johns Hopkins Press, 1985.

Olsen J, Trichopoulos D, eds. *Teaching Epidemiology: What You Should Know and What You Could Do.* Oxford, New York, Melbourne: Oxford Medical Publications, 1992.

Patrick DL, Erickson P. *Health Status and Health Policy.* New York: Oxford University Press, 1993.

Petitti DB. *Meta-Analysis, Decision Analysis, and Cost-Effectiveness Analysis: Methods for Quantitative Synthesis in Medicine.* New York: Oxford University Press, 1994.

Rothman KJ. *Modern Epidemiology.* Boston: Little, Brown, 1986.

Rothman KJ, ed. *Causal Inference.* Chestnut Hill, MA: Epidemiology Resources, 1988.

Sackett DL, Haynes RB, Tugwell P. *Clinical Epidemiology,* 2nd ed. Boston: Little, Brown, 1992.

Schlesselman JJ. *Case-Control Studies: Design, Conduct, Analysis.* New York: Oxford University Press, 1982.

Silverman WA. *Human Experimentation: A Guided Step into the Unknown.* Oxford, London, New York: Oxford University Press, 1985.

Susser MW. *Causal Thinking in the Health Sciences.* New York: Oxford University Press, 1973.

Susser MW. *Epidemiology, Health and Society: Selected Papers.* New York: Oxford University Press, 1987.

Swaroop S. *Introduction to Health Statistics.* Edinburgh: Livingstone, 1960.

Teutsch SM, Churchill RE. *Principles and Practice of Public Health Surveillance.* New York: Oxford University Press, 1994.

US Preventive Services Task Force. *Guide to Clinical Preventive Services.* Baltimore, MD: Williams & Wilkins, 1989.

Works of historical interest, and the history of epidemiology

Buck C, Llopis A, Nájera E, Terris M, eds. *The Challenge of Epidemiology: Issues and Selected Readings.* Washington, DC: Pan American Health Organization, 1988.

Farr W. *Vital Statistics: A Memorial Volume of Selections from the Reports and Writings of William Farr.* Edited by Noel Humphries. London: Stanford, 1985. (Revised, edited, and annotated edition introduced by MW Susser and A Adelstein, published under the auspices of the New York Academy of Medicine, 1975.)

Greenland S, ed. *Evolution of Epidemiologic Ideas: Annotated Readings on Concepts and Methods.* Chestnut Hill, MA: Epidemiology Resources, 1987.

Greenwood M. *Epidemics and Crowd Diseases: An Introduction to the Study of Epidemiology.* London: Williams and Norgate, 1935.

Hamer W. *Epidemiology Old and New.* London: Kegan Paul, 1928.

Snow J. *On the Mode of Communication of Cholera,* 2nd ed, much enlarged. London: Churchill, 1855. Reprinted in *Snow on Cholera,* edited by WH Frost, with a biographical memoir by BW Richardson. New York: Commonwealth Fund, 1936. Reprinted 1965, New York: Hafner.

Stallybrass CO. *The Principles of Epidemiology.* London: Routledge, 1931.

White KL, Frenk J, Ordóñez C, et al, eds. *Health Services Research: An Anthology.* Washington, DC: Pan American Health Organization, 1992.

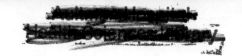